Runner's World

MASSAGE BOOK

Runner's World

MASSAGE BOOK

by Ray Hosler

Illustrations
by David Hebenstreit

Runner's World Books

Library of Congress Cataloging in Publication Data

Hosler, Ray, 1952-
    Runner's World massage book.

    Runner's World books.
    1. Massage. I. Runner's World. II. Title.
III. Title: Massage book.
RM721.H64   615.8'22   82-5304
ISBN 0-89037-229-2 (spiral) AACR 2
ISBN 0-89037-240-3 (perfectbound)
ISBN 0-89037-252-7 (hardbound)

2nd printing May, 1983

Contents

Acknowledgments. vi
Dedication. vii
Introduction ix
Massage Through the Ages. 1
There is a Massage for You 11
Life at a Massage Center 43
A Full-Body Experience 59
Body Maintenance. 67
Lotions and Potions 103
Learning the Techniques. 107
Laying of the Hands 113
Massage for the Young and Elderly. 179
Massage for the Athlete. 185
Glossary 193
Bibliography 205
About the Author 207
Recommended Reading. 209

Acknowledgments

The following individuals have been particularly helpful in lending their expertise and in giving advice for the book. They are: Robin Tobias, who, along with Linda Chrisman, describes the massage process in Chapter 8. Robin appears in the photos in Chapter 8, also; Marcia Nelson and Michael Murphy, for answering my interview questions, however dumb they might have seemed; Dave Hebenstreit, for his excellent drawings; Betty Fuller (Trager), Helga Brandt (Touch for Health) and Janet Loops (Feldenkrais), for providing information or demonstrating their respective bodywork practices; Sarah Seemans for describing massage for the elderly, Deane Juhan, for his analysis of massage at Esalen; Mark Sisson, for receiving the massage in Chapter 8 (he needed it after his fourth-place finish in the Hawaii Iron Man Triathlon); David Keith, for taking the photos in Chapter 8; and Doris Sukinikie, physical therapist at The Midpeninsula Health Center in Palo Alto, California, who made my neck better.

Dedication

To my family and friends

Introduction

Most of the books on massage have been written by experienced practitioners who know their subject from the inside out. The reader and the profession obviously benefit from this point of view. The reader gets the inside story and members of the profession see different ways to apply their work.

Occasionally, however, a profession and its members can benefit from the views of someone from the outside, such as myself—a professional journalist. My perspectives will, hopefully, cast a new light on the subject of massage while being informative and entertaining. Many readers will be looking into massage for the first time and to be able to read from the consumer's point of view should prove helpful. Over the past six months I have interviewed and received various forms of massage and bodywork from more than a dozen practitioners, and in the accumulation of information I have discovered that each practitioner has his or her unique style for working the body. Even with Swedish massage, which has a well-systematized set of strokes and techniques and has been practiced for centuries, there are differences from one practitioner to the next.

Most of you are obviously aware that there is legitimate and illegitimate massage available in this country. Massage parlors fall into the category of illegitimate and are merely covers for prostitution. This unfortunate choice of words—massage parlor—was coined only in the last two decades, but it quickly took the profession's reputation from its place in physical therapy and health clubs to the depths of human decadence. But with the sexual revolution of the 1960s, which spawned massage parlors, there also evolved a group of individuals who recognized massage as clean, healthful and an integral part of holistic health. They saw massage as sensual, not necessarily sexual.

Holistic health is perhaps the best of the health trends that has come the way of American society in the last century. It has yet to spread throughout the country and to gain full acceptance in all medical circles, but holistic health and the lifestyle it encourages is here to stay. Too many people have discovered its benefits to let it die now. Were Americans to practice it, the cure for cancer that science seeks and spends so many millions of dollars on annually might not be such a fervent goal. Together, holistic health and preventive medicine can do more to combat cancer and other debilitating diseases than any drug medical science might come up with.

Holism, from which the word holistic is derived, can be defined as the view that an organic or integrated whole has a reality independent of and greater than the sum of its parts. The connotations here are clearly spiritual, but holistic health is grounded in common sense principles—there is no religion to follow, no group that must be joined, no communion that should be practiced. To be holistic is to realize that everything you do in life has some affect on both your mind and body. When you consume alcohol it not only dulls the brain but it changes body chemistry. When you become physically active you not only improve the body but make your mind more alert. And, just as there is a physical side to life, there is also a spiritual side, however you may view it.

American society is an adaptive one—it accepts many different beliefs and peoples—and that is an important asset today, since social norms, the very basis for providing structure and cohesion in our lives, themselves have been ripped from their moorings and set adrift in the currents of change. The family, which has held together every important civilization and has served as the foundation of love and communication among peoples, has faced a severe test the past several decades from an increasingly automated lifestyle. Even in tradition-bound China where families routinely trace their roots over more than a millenium, the recent influence of Western thought and values has caused some stress. Today, divorce, once unheard of in China, is on the increase in the capital, Peking, which has received the strongest dose of Western influence. Paradoxically, the state of California, which has led our nation in divorce, recently showed a decrease in its rate over the past several years. It remains to be seen if this is just a lull, an aberrant trend, or a sign of some lasting shift back to traditional patterns.

This love and compassion once so easily obtained from family and friends is now not so easy to come by. Now there is social unrest. Some families have literally been cast to the winds by this mobile world in which travel between continents is as easy as stepping on a jet plane for a journey that lasts mere hours. Traditional role playing is being questioned by both sexes, causing uncertainty, suspicion and divisions that have gone so far as to generate the popular concept of women's liberation and the petition for a new amendment to the Constitution.

During unsettled times we instinctively reach out for something —a belief or a concept or a religion or a physical object—anything that will give us some sense of security and permanence. Some of us find this security in holding a good job or buying as many material goods as we can afford. Others seek emotional well-being through a lasting relationship. However, these ideal relationships have become increasingly difficult to establish, so alternatives are developing that encourage satisfaction through different means. Here is where massage and bodywork have found their place in our society and will continue to expand.

Showing interest for another person can be expressed in many forms other than sexual. And we all crave attention. For example, getting a haircut at a barber shop is relaxing, pleasant and a simple form of therapy. Here is someone who cares about you. The barber trims your hair, he prunes it, runs his comb through it—he pampers you. He works around the sensitive neck and sometimes the brush of a hand against the skin feels soothing. Your friendly barber serves as a down-home psychologist, too, taking in all your day-to-day concerns, almost always agreeing with you and offering words of encouragement.

A massage follows the same idea as sitting in the barber's chair, but the results and the relationship between the client and practitioner are more far-reaching. For one hour you are receiving attention from someone's caring hands. You can discuss problems with your practitioner just as you would with your barber; he or she will give encouragement and support. And you are able to let go of some of your pent-up frustrations.

While the benefits of massage in terms of emotional well-being have been stressed, we cannot ignore the positive physical effects. Many of the new bodywork systems are proving to have tremendous benefits for rehabilitation from injuries, muscle imbalances, even emotional problems. For years chiropractic and osteopathy were the only sources of non-standard medical care available, but that has changed. This is not to say that chiropractic and osteopathy are no longer available, just that there are now alternatives. If chiropractic can't fix your back maybe Aston-Patterning can.

Finally, there is monetary cost involved in having any massage or bodywork done by a professional, and that is bound to influence your decision about getting treatment. The cost ranges from $20 to $40 an hour. It has always been the nature of people to forego medical treatment for financial reasons, much less any kind of care outside of traditional medical circles, so there is going to be some resistance until a greater percentage of the public experiences a sensual massage and the word spreads.

For now, the financial burden rests with the individual and you must decide whether or not the thirty dollars you spend on a new pair of shoes will go instead to an hour of massage. The intent of this book is to say to the public that there is good in massage, for the body and soul, and that it has intrinsic value. Touching is a primary cohesive force between members of the human race.

It has been said that life is a feast; if you think this is true, then massage is your dessert. Enjoy.

1

Massage Through the Ages

Massage has a written history spanning nearly 5000 years and has influenced all of the world's great civilizations. It is a history of man's joys, his self-discovery and, occasionally, his repression. Evolving from the rudimentary touch to an accepted art form, in liberal times it flourished, as with the Greeks and Romans, but in conservative eras it was repressed, as with the Victorian Age. It even fell into camp with Satanism in the European Dark Ages. Its message and implementation has followed two distinctly different paths—for healing and for enjoyment. While massage quickly found a place the world over as a pleasurable activity, its acceptance by the modern medical and therapeutic fields has been much slower. But it appears we are now seeing that what we thought were two divergent paths of massage are really the same, that one does not occur without the other. From the beginning, man rubbed his wounds for therapy and mothers carressed their children for pleasure.

Massage became popular well before the time of the powerful Greek city states, which produced one of the most significant advances in human knowledge; its Western roots extend to the ancient Egyptians and Mesopotamians, whose public baths served as venues for taking in an afternoon massage under the sun. In the Far East, too, massage has enjoyed a long and popular following. As early as 3000 B.C., books were written about massage, to describe what had already become an art among the Chinese and Japanese. *Cong-Fou of the Tao-Tse*, the oldest known book written about massage, gave the West many of its techniques. French scholars translated the book in the 18th century and it served as a foundation for the modern European massage that was systematized by the Swedes and Germans.

Our first accounts of massage in the Western world originate from the Greeks and Romans, whose rich heritage was meticulously recorded and has been preserved through the centuries. Greek physicians, while breaking ground for modern Western medicine, found massage beneficial to their patients' health, so much so that they compelled them to have their bodies "rubbed." These doctors followed the way of the famous Greek physician Herodicus (c. 500 B.C., and not to be confused with Heroditus, the father of history), who prescribed a simple form of gymnastics for his healing patients. He is considered the originator of medical gymnastics, an early branch of massage popular in the 18th and 19th centuries. Medical gymnastics exercises were quite similar to the present-day movements taught in our public schools —jumping jacks, sit-ups, push-ups, and so on.

Hippocrates (c. 460 B.C.-c. 370 B.C.), the Greek physician considered the father of medicine, also believed in recommending massage to his patients. He said that physicians should be experienced in rubbing, "for things that have the same name have not always the same effect. Rubbing can bind a joint that is too loose, and loosen a joint that is too rigid. Rubbing can make flesh, and cause parts to waste." For treating a separated shoulder he said, "And it is necessary to rub the shoulder gently and smoothly. However, a shoulder in the condition described should be rubbed with soft hands and above all things gently; the joint should be moved about not violently, but so far as it can be done without producing pain."

Hippocrates coined massage "anatripsis," Greek for friction. He directed that friction should be applied centripetally, or in the direction blood flows in the veins, thus demonstrating his understanding of the circulatory system and how massage plays an active role in improving circulation. Hippocrates, who learned massage and medical gymnastics from Herodicus, also said of massage, "Friction can relax, brace, incarnate [fleshen] and attenuate; hard braces, soft relaxes, much attenuates and moderate thickens."

Healing through massage was held in such high regard by the Greeks that Asclepiades of Bithynia (c. 124 B.C.-40 B.C.), the founder of an influential school of medicine in Rome, abandoned the use of all medicines, relying exclusively on massage, which he claimed effects a cure by restoring the nutritive fluids their natural, free movement. He postulated that disease is caused by disturbances in the movements of atoms or particles, of which he believed the body was composed.

Massage represents one aspect of the Ancient Greeks fascination with the human body and mind. Long-held and inaccurate beliefs about human anatomy, such as the aorta transporting oxygen, rather than blood, fell to the wayside as Greek physicians began probing and dissecting (some scholars argue that the Greeks did not dissect). But technology was still far too primitive to open doors to cures for most diseases and ailments, so massage found a place in medicine. It was easy to do and made the patient feel better—for whatever reason—even though it might not have cured him. The tide has since changed, however, as pills and complex machines used in medicine and physical therapy today usually supplant the slower, more mundane, but much more humane massage.

Massage took a more pleasurable slant with the Romans, reaching its apex of decadence under Caesar (c. 102 B.C.-44 B.C.), perhaps the most controversial ruler of the vast Roman Empire. Hollywood movies had a hand in showing the stereotypical massage setting—one of toga-robed Romans gathered around marble baths that overlook the Mediterranean Sea. Caesar's personal council, surrounded by a contingent of beautiful female slaves, was waited on hand and foot and given regular massages. This much-idealized scene was not without truth, however. Caesar played court with his loyal politicians by seeing that they lived stylishly: Roman baths, beautiful women and a free massage were rewards for loyalty to the emperor. Massage also had a special place with Caesar, because it gave him relief from neuralgia and epileptic seizures.

Perhaps this Hollywood-fostered image of the Roman baths and massage for the rich has added to the decadent tone enveloping the art. Mention having a "massage" today and immediately your friends envision something sensuous, something sexy and definitely something very enjoyable.

Even as the Roman baths overflowed with patrons who were there to receive a massage, its medical use continued with the Roman physicians. Aulus Cornelius Celsus, Roman leader in the field of medicine at the beginning of the Christian era, used massage extensively. He recommended manipulations of the head for the relief of headaches and general manipulations to restore the surface circulation in fever, saying, "A patient is in bad shape when the exterior of the body is cold, the interior hot with thirst; but, indeed, also, the only safeguard lies in rubbing." Celsus also used a sort of percussion, called whipping, in treating disease. In another, more deadly arena, massage found a place. Galen (c. 130 A.D.-200 A.D.), physician to the School of Gladiators at Pergamum, ordered the bodies of the combatants to be rubbed until "they were red and anointed" to prepare for the "exercises." Obviously, this massage loosened the gladiators' muscles so that they would not be stiff when combat ensued. The same idea applies to track and field athletes who massage before competition, only in this case they are rubbing down to avoid muscle pulls and not the sword of some opposing gladiator. Sprinters, especially, need to be massaged before competition because they are placing instant and severe demands on leg muscles.

Many ideas the Greeks and Romans developed about massage came from observing animals. Around the time of the Christian era the Greek historian Arian chronicled his observations on massage for animals. He claimed that massage strengthened their limbs, rendered their hair soft and glossy and cleansed the skin of horses and dogs. After giving directions for massaging the legs, abdomen and back, he directed that the treatment of a dog be terminated in the following peculiar manner: "Lift her up by the tail and give her a good stretching; let her go and she will shake herself and show that she liked the treatment." Arian was practicing a technique called nerve stretching.

Whereas the Greeks had good reason to believe that massage could actually cure disease (What better method was there at the time?), by the Middle Ages medical knowledge had advanced enough so that physicians knew its power to heal was limited. They began seeing it as an adjunct to treatment, rather than a cure-all. Massage could no more *cure* epilepsy than could faith healing cure cancer. However, there were still those who believed that massage, like faith healing, had a mystical power—the power of touch. Hartvig Nissen writes in *Practical Massage and Corrective Exercises*, "Many a poor woman was burned at the stake in northern Europe during the Middle Ages because she knew little more than other persons and cured suffering men by massage, a magic which was looked upon as the power of Satan." How times have changed.

Europe renewed its interest in massage during the 16th and 18th centuries, with the translation of many Chinese and Greek writings. Physicians still used massage and so, too, were rulers receiving it. Friedrich Hoffman (1660-1742), physician to the King of Prussia around 1700, recommended rubbing and exercises (medical gymnastics) for the royal court, as did many physicians in Scandinavia, France and England.

English essayist Lord Francis Bacon (1561-1626), one of the era's greatest statesmen and scientists, made this telling observation about massage: "Frictions make the parts more fleshy and full, as we see both in men and the carrying of the horses. The cause is for that they draw greater quantity of spirits and blood to the parts and again because they draw the ailments more forcibly from within, and again because they relax the pores and so make the better passage of the spirits, blood and ailment; lastly because they dissipate and digest any inutile and excrementitious moisture, which lieth in the flesh, all which helps assimilation." Bacon shows his keen understanding of how massage benefits the body, which shows how medical science and the scientific method had advanced since the Ancient Greeks.

Oriental massage techniques, especially those of the Japanese, found a receptive audience in Europe and their methods served as the foundation for much of Swedish massage. One Oriental translation of the 19th century is told in *The Art of Massage*, a book by John Harvey Kellogg. According to an associate of Kellogg's, the Japanese employed, almost exclusively, blind men or women for conducting massage. These blind practitioners would go about the streets soliciting patients in a loud voice, yelling "Amma!

Kellogg's account of massage is given by the associate, who sought out one of these practitioners to relieve his cold and fever:

"The shampooer [shampoo is from the Hindi, meaning "press"] sat in Japanese fashion at the side of the patient, as the latter lay on a futon (thick comforter or quilt) on the floor, and began operations on the arm; then took the back and the back of the neck, afterward the head (top and forehead) and ended with the legs. On the arms, back, back of the neck, and legs, he used sometimes the tips of his fingers, sometimes the palms or the backs of his hands, sometimes his knuckles, sometimes his fists. The movements consisted of pinching, slapping, stroking, rubbing, knuckling, kneading, thumping, drawing in the hand, and snapping the knuckles. The rubbing in the vicinity of the ribs was slightly ticklish and the knuckling on the back of neck and the side of the collarbone, a little painful. On the head he used gentle tapping, a little pounding with the knuckles, stroking with both hands, holding the head tight for a moment, grasping it with one hand and stroking it with the other. The operator seemed to have a good practical knowledge of physiology and anatomy, and certainly succeeded in driving away the headache and languor, in producing a pleasant tingling throughout the body, and in restoring normal circulation of the blood . . ."

Even a century later this description might apply, when you consider that techniques haven't changed all that much.

While the Japanese refined massage techniques learned from the Chinese, Europeans pushed ahead to give massage its deserved place in physical therapy. The key name linked to the transition of massage from heresay to scientific documentation is that of Peter Henry Ling (1776-1839), who was instrumental in carrying through the establishment of the Royal Gymnastic Institute, in Stockholm, Sweden, in 1813. This was the first college for pedagogical, military and medical gymnastics and it was here that Ling finalized his teachings to a format we know today as Swedish massage, a catch-all for many different massage techniques, and still the best known massage in the West. Ling did not originate the Swedish movements; he merely systematized them. Ling, formerly a gymnast instructor and champion fencer, took special interest in the recuperative power of massage and exercise after it helped cure him of rheumatism in the arm.

R. Mezger of Amsterdam carried on with the advancement of massage as a form of physical therapy in the late 19th century through his success in treating the Danish Crown Prince, who suffered from a chronic joint affection. Mezger won the confidence of the public and high officials and exerted powerful influence upon the study of massage by the medical world.

Medical gymnastics had its greatest influence in the 19th century and its success was due in part to the industrial revolution. With all the foundries busting at the seams to make new products, it is not entirely surprising that they contributed to the medical field. Some bizarre-looking contraptions came into use for physical therapy—medical gymnastics—which, even if they didn't succeed in their design, no doubt impressed the patients (some favorably and some not so favorably) who used them. The West was just beginning to benefit from the advent of machinery, so the public must have truly believed that these complex mechanical devices were going to help them cure their ills. Most of the machinery consisted of wheels, gears and pulleys, all to stretch the muscles in the body or to manipulate them in various ways.

It was bad enough that the physical therapist's rehabilitation facility looked like a chamber of horrors, but the sad fact was that getting a massage from your friendly doctor back then was no treat. The basic theory held by medical minds then said that if it was to get better it would have to hurt. And it did. If sado-masochism wasn't a major theme of the Victorian Era, it would be hard to find any other reason for some of the treatment forms used in physical therapy. One procedure called for the patient to hang by his hands from a crossbar. While suspended in midair he was pushed, shoved and hit by his therapist, the same way a punching bag gets batted around by a boxer in training. Books published on physical therapy showing such brutality have long since gone out of print and so have the practices, but some of the photos are reprinted in *The Art of Sensual Massage*, authored by Gordon Inkeles. Inkeles is by no means recommending such treat-ment; the photos are merely in a section of his book, published in 1972, dealing with the history of massage.

To explain why massage became so mechanical and unemotion-al during the Victorian Age you also have to look at the social ethics and morals of the time. Queen Victoria, who ruled England longer than any previous royalty (over sixty years), was a strict disciplinarian with equally high moral values. She expected her fellow countrymen to follow in her righteous footsteps, although it is interesting to note that she married her own cousin and had nine children by him. This puritan ethic from England made its way to America and dominated throughout the 19th century, and perhaps that is why few publications on massage emerged at this time. It was Douglas Graham, a Boston physician, who first came out with significant information on massage in Amer-ica, in *Practical Treatise on Massage.* By the early part of the 20th century more books became available; however, they dealt almost exclusively with medical gymnastics.

Massage as a sensual art didn't find its place in this country until the early 1960s, interestingly, about the time our sexual values also began to take a more "liberal" course. Previous to that, physical therapists continued with their scientific analysis of the effects of massage. They went to great lengths, measuring blood circulation, taking body temperatures before and after massage, even conducting a stomach massage on the top of Pikes Peak, a 14,000-foot mountain in the Colorado Rockies. This was the age of the scientific method. It was also a time when physical therapy schools adopted Albert J. Hoffa's style of massage, based on his *Technik der Massage*, published in 1900 in Germany.

Massage has taken its more sensual course, a means of physical and spiritual fulfillment, only in the last twenty years. With the drug generation, the rock and roll generation, the sexual revolution generation came the "sensual massage" generation. Inkeles writes in *The Art of Sensual Massage,* ". . . you can use your hands to bring immense pleasure to another human being without the coldness of traditional therapy and outside the intimacies of sex. There is a wide spectrum of human feeling between the poles of therapy and sex—we call it sensual."

You first have to break down the sexual taboos built up over the past century in America; it requires a liberal attitude and a spirit of understanding and cooperation.

Nowhere is massage as a sensual art form more prevalent than in California. California is a liberal enclave for almost every form of spiritual and social enlightenment known to man, accepting the religions of the Far East and the most radical lifestyles devised by some of this country's greatest and most innovative thinkers. It was in California that Esalen took root and flourished to become a clearing house for new massage techniques. It was in California that two of the most popular massage books' authors learned and wrote about sensual massage. *The Massage Book* by George Downing and *The Art of Sensual Massage* by Gordon Inkeles, both published in 1972, have been the trend-setters for published material on massage. Their books have combined sales of over one million copies, so it is apparent that we have taken to sensual massage with zeal, and there are literally hundreds of massage centers throughout California now, with schools and institutes devoted to a vast array of techniques. And there is no shortage of patrons.

Massage has also become a convenient cover for prostitution— much to the distress of the sensual school of thought—in the form of massage parlors. According to Peter Whittaker, author of *The American Way of Sex*, they got their sordid start in 1972 when an ad in *Screw* magazine, a New York underground sex publication, offered "Private Body-Painting Sessions." Of course, it was a shallow ploy for the "legal" buying and selling of sex and from that obscure beginning massage parlors have spread like a malignant cancer to every large city across the United States. There is no shortage of masseuses and masseurs either, when you consider that their salaries can run as high as $2000 a week and that there is little chance of them being caught for their victimless crimes. Obviously, massage parlors are not places to go for a sensual massage and it shouldn't be very hard to pick out one business from another. If you have any concerns about the legitimacy of a massage business, just call your local health care center or the police department; they'll be able to give you their opinion.

What of the future of massage? According to one massage practitioner, it all depends on the political climate of the time. As long as the liberal aspects of society exist, massage will flourish. Right now it appears that massage may be enjoying its greatest fling since the days of the Roman baths, much to our good fortune.

2

There is a Massage for You

You might not think that the activity of rubbing another person's body could have so many different forms that it is considered an art, but the variety you have in which to choose from is astonishing. Some methods originate in the Far East and have thousand-year histories, while others are born in the last two decades of the recent wave of psycho-physical therapy. A practice may be universal, as with Swedish massage, or limited to a small following. Most of the massage forms listed here can be enjoyable, but there are some that fall in the gray area, between painful physical therapy and sensual massage, such as rolfing. At times some rolfers will apply considerable pressure and there may be a variety of other unusual sensations experienced, in rolfing, and other massage forms. I have been liberal in the definition of a massage technique. In the strictest sense some of the following methods would be considered bodywork and not massage; however, in order to provide as many different systems as possible, the boundaries of definition have been stretched. The basic premise is that each method here involves touching another person for the purpose of either providing enjoyment or as a healing process removed from textbook physical therapy. Because a massage technique is little understood and has a limited audience does not mean that it will languish forever, nor should it if it can be of aid to mankind. Remember that Chinese acupuncture is still a mystery to Western scientists, although its use is becoming increasingly popular here, especially as a form of anesthesia. Less than a decade ago most doctors had labeled acupuncture "quackupuncture."

You are responsible for choosing the massage that best suits your needs and desires. Don't always choose a massage by what your friends recommend, either. Their reaction to a massage may be completely different from yours. No two people respond to touch in the same way. Some prefer a light stroke, while others will want to experience kneading and friction. That's because we all have different thresholds of pain, as well as preconceived notions as to what we find pleasurable. You also have to consider your mood at the time of the massage; have you had a recent traumatic experience that will put you in a different "head space"? Or are you feeling particularly good? Certain massage techniques call for the right state of mind and if you're not feeling that way you may not enjoy the massage as much as you had anticipated.

Atmosphere is as important as your state of mind, so you should know where you feel comfortable, because not all massage centers will appeal to your senses, for reasons ranging from background noise, the kind of music played or the lighting used. It also seems that with each technique there is a slightly different setting that a particular practitioner likes to work in or feels most effective with. Many of the decisions we make about a situation, in terms of good or bad, are in fact the result of how we react to our environment, so be aware.

Perhaps as important as the massage you find comfortable is to locate a practitioner who you can enjoy being with. A good practitioner is critical; inexperienced practitioners or veterans who don't have the right touch, can turn a potentially rewarding hour into a nightmare, leaving you tense and with more sore muscles than you had when you started. From the beginning, you must decide who you will feel more comfortable with, a masseur or a masseuse. Their manner of speech, dress and especially touch is obviously important. One masseur, as a way of making his clients feel more comfortable, wears a long skirt and he says that it is an amazingly effective method; however, you will be surprised to find that most practitioners dress quite conservatively.

Finally, there is an intangible factor that cannot be measured on a ruler or weighed on a scale in choosing a masseur; that's because this criteria has to do with energy vibrations. We can't see them, we can't touch them but they're there, just as there is a magnetic field between the poles of the earth. Our energy field varies with the emotional and physical state we're in. When we are feeling healthy and happy we emit good vibrations. We gain a better understanding of another person's energy field the better we know them. We can sense their moods and act accordingly. Touching another person is one method of picking up their strongest vibrations and the manner in which we touch that person, including the kind of feelings we are emitting, can influence another.

When a practitioner touches you, that very subtle energy transfer takes place. Your reaction could be neutral, positive or negative. You know when you've found that right practitioner, though, when his movements seem to fall into place with your desires; this harmony is no less powerful than a symphony orchestra giving a great performance of Beethoven's "Fifth Symphony." Time flies during the massage and you wish it would never end as you and the masseur link up. Finding the right practitioner is another matter; it could take time and some searching. Your closest friend probably has the right wavelength—otherwise you wouldn't be so close—but how good is he or she at giving a massage?

The following are some of the better-known systems of touching and some of the not so well known. There are literally hundreds of new massage forms springing up around the country, with strange names, strange ideas and some techniques that feel quite unusual. You'll also discover a considerable overlap between techniques and that many of their goals are practically identical. I have tried to include only the most important systems today and some of the newer methods that appear to have considerable promise for becoming much more popular than they are.

SWEDISH

It came to the Western world by way of the Far East and then through medical gymnastics. Like so many massage forms, Swedish technique varies from practitioner to practitioner; however, the methods used today can be traced for the most part to the German Albert Hoffa and his therapeutic massage methods, which employ stroking, friction, kneading, percussion and so on.

Swedish massage gained widespread popularity in the United States right after World War I, for the rehabilitation of veterans. Physical therapists were becoming an increasingly important asset to hospitals and they were in turn using massage with considerable success. By the 1930s every major hospital staffed physical therapists, who were using massage on a regular basis. It was no coincidence that health clubs began using Swedish massage just as it was becoming popular for medical purposes. Health club owners were the first to witness the influx of injured veterans intent on using their facilities for rehabilitation (with weights, stationary bikes, swimming pools, saunas, etc.) and the owners quickly added training masseurs to their staffs to lure in more customers in need of rehabilitative massage.

Everyone is probably familiar with the stereotyped Swedish massage scene that takes place in the local health club. A heavyset masseur hacks, slaps and pounds on an overweight patron, who has just emerged from a steam bath and has a towel wrapped around his waist. He lies down on a table covered with white sheets and tries to relax. The masseur is a gruff sort of fellow — really a nice guy once you get to know him—with huge, hairy arms that look like they could snap telephone poles in half; you don't want to rile him during the massage. By the time the massage is over, the patron gets slowly up from the table, not sure whether he has just been mugged or had a healthful, relaxing massage, as he was expecting. The masseur then slaps him on the back, smiles, and with a gleam in his eyes says, "See you next week!"

You can still re-enact this situation in many health clubs, the ones with the old-timer who will talk your ear off about the World Series or the upcoming Super Bowl. But many of the new health clubs have a more sophisticated, better-educated masseur; he may even have considerable knowledge of sports kinesiology. He could probably take care of your sports injury as well as anyone, but if you're looking for a soothing, enjoyable massage in a relaxed setting, you'll probably have to go elsewhere. On the other hand, if you want to talk baseball while downing a beer or two, and this is what you consider relaxation, the health spa masseur may be just the person you're looking for.

Swedish massage, in many different varieties, is also offered at most massage centers. If you ask for a Swedish massage you will most likely find a relaxed atmosphere, and receive lots of stroking, kneading and some occasional friction. How much you enjoy it depends largely on how good your practitioner is at using the various techniques, which are described in Chapter 7.

ESALEN

Esalen Institute is "a center to explore those trends in education, religion, philosophy, and the physical and behavorial sciences which emphasize the potentialities and values of human existence," as stated on the back of its catalog. This human-potential foundation gained impetus in the turbulent decade of the 1960s, a time when America's youth were discovering the real world, their real selves and the new reality of how life must be lived in the nuclear age. Their world, our world, is one in which disease has been all but wiped out and basic necessities are readily met, but the constant threat of world annihilation clouds the future of man.

Esalen became an instrument for sifting through the wealth of ideas and information that can help us survive the coming decades. Its activities now include seminars and workshops (anywhere from two days to one month in length), residential programs, consulting and research. Massage is but one of the workshops offered.

As for Esalen massage itself, the name implies many concepts but not a specific technique with respect to how the hands are used or the way in which a body is manipulated. To gain further insight into Esalen and how it became so closely associated with massage, Deane Juhan, an eight-year staff member of Esalen, gives his views and insights into Esalen and massage. Juhan attended the University of California at Berkeley, English literature graduate school, before moving to Esalen, and has never looked back. "I left school and got into massage as a way to get over my shyness," he explains. Here is his analysis of Esalen and massage:

"The genre name, Esalen massage, shows up everywhere but here. People use that as an advertisement for doing some kind of massage work. I don't know what they do, but most of the advertisers who I've seen using that word are people who have never been here or nobody here has ever heard of them.

"We have a unique situation here. There is no one person who holds the keys and tells everyone what to do. It's been a very long, democratic, exploratory process over eighteen years and probably thirty major people contributing. When Esalen was founded about eighteen years ago it became something more than just a lodge and an inn where people could come down [from the San Francisco Bay Area] for the weekend. It started to become a therapy center, a growth center. A man named Bernie Gunther first trained people here to do massage work. He had a small staff and some of the original people here do massage work. He used a Swedish massage mixture from several different schools of thought, but the underlying philosophy was a gentling, nurturing, mothering, stroking, soft massage. It was not designed necessarily to stimulate your capillaries or align your bones or necessarily do any of those therapeutic things. It was supposed to be a safe, non-sexual, sensual bath that carried the same mood of the safe environment of the work group they were in at the time. That was really the therapy—the massage—giving people that peace, that calm and relaxation.

"I think that philosophical core has in many ways held on. I think if there's a psychological, therapeutic core to what everybody does here it's that—creating a situation of trust, a psychological situation of peace and release and the feeling that anything that comes up you can talk about. We can deal with it. Not so much, 'Okay, we're going to fix your knee. Now lie down and turn it three degrees to the right while I do this and that.' Now what's happened on top of that basic idea is that for the past years the people who Bernie trained went their various ways and new people came in with new methods. All of us worked together and we all (not as a group) had training from many different people. We've had several people who have gone to rolfing school. We have a small offshoot of rolfing taught by Al Decker (one of Ida's first students) called deep tissue. The Rolfing Institute used to be here before it moved to Boulder, Colorado. The first trainings by Ida were done here.

"The long and short of what I'm saying is that just about every major influence that you can think of that has happened in the last ten years has found its way in here through one practitioner or another.

"Part of the power of what our crew manages to get down here has to do with how tremendously peaceful and beautiful the surroundings are. On a day like today, when it's a nice day, I'm working up on top of a deck that's about 100 feet over the Pacific Ocean and you can look straight down into the surf. There's a little cove, so you're surrounded by cliffs and the sun's spilling down. We do our massage work among concrete and cinder bathhouses that face the ocean. There are hot springs here open to the public, but on a restricted schedule." Esalen Foundation is about thirty miles south of Monterey Bay, in the heart of Los Padres National Forest in central California.

"I think there are two basic things Esalen has contributed to the massage movement over the years. One is the development of a style itself that has to do with Esalen and the Esalen style of bodywork. I think it has really disseminated itself widely so that a lot of people come here and see that is what they want. A lot of practitioners come down and take our workshops to get a view through a different window of what they're doing.

"And the other is that this is a kind of Ed Sullivan Show for anybody who's got a new technique. It's really the showcase of virtually every technique that comes down the road."

To learn more about Esalen you can write to Esalen Institute, Big Sur, California 93920.

ROLFING

It sounds a bit odd, and, well, it is. Rolfing is one of those modern-day procedures of body manipulation aimed at bringing the body into proper alignment. Not so strange. It's strangeness is in the execution, to be described later.

Rolfing is named for its creator, Dr. Ida P. Rolf (her Ph.D. was in biological chemistry), from whom many current practitioners learned her methods. The technical name is Structural Integration, but became known as rolfing at Esalen, where Dr. Rolf perfected her system. She began rolfing by using it on herself and her sickly son; Dr. Rolf had arthritis. She died in 1980, at the age of eighty-four. Her practice has long since gained a dedicated following and there is a national rolf institute in Boulder, Colorado.

Dr. Rolf based her philosophy of rolfing on monism. Monism, basically, is the belief that one thing, or object, or god, or influence rules our lives and affects everything we do. The Christian faith is monistic because it recognizes only one god.

If you believe that all mental and physical actions of the body are interrelated then you are monistic. The opposite theory, dualism, has been the foundation of Western thought since the Ancient Greeks, who determined that the universe can be divided into energy and matter.

Dr. Rolf believed that the human body is monistic in that everything that happens to us, whether it be mental or physical, affects us both mentally and physically. Her reasoning is best illustrated with a scenario: Let's say a child falls out of his crib. He immediately begins crying and screaming. Mother comes and picks baby up. Initially nothing appears to be wrong with the baby, other than a bruise. Just to be sure, mother takes baby to her pediatrician for a checkup. The doctor finds everything normal and mother breathes a sigh of relief. But unknown to doctor and mother, baby has a damaged hip joint. By grade-school age the boy has trouble running and does poorly in sports. He withdraws from outdoor activities and becomes increasingly moody. A picture of discontent forms and the groundwork for future emotional problems is laid. Admittedly, this is simplistic reasoning; however, the point is that mental and physical events interact.

So much for the philosophy of rolfing. Its intent is to realign the body (the hip joint in the case of the baby)—to bring about structural integration through the manual manipulation of the fascia. Structural integration is the reordering of the body by bringing the major segments—head, shoulders, thorax, pelvis and the legs—toward a vertical alignment. In other words, having good posture. Probably nine out of ten bodies are out of whack in one way or another because most of us have taken a fall at one time, say from a bicycle. You may have limped around for a while and within the next couple of months regained full mobility. But most likely there has been some form of muscle compensation; perhaps one calf muscle takes more strain than the other. The fascia, the interconnective tissue, is also placed under stress and it in turn gives your body a subtly different posture.

The rolfer's job is to rebalance the fascial network by taking advantage of the body's tendency to hold the shapes induced by an applied force. The rolfer must move the tissue back toward the body's proper balance, similar to a mechanic bending the bent frame of a bicycle to make it rideable. Rolfers work on the fascia, a fibrous membrane covering, supporting and separating muscle. Deep fascia, when traumatized, or inflamed by illness, can cause surrounding structures and muscles to adhere to one another. Consider the whiplash victim. Months after the accident his neck is still sore and stiff because of tight muscles and a buildup of scar tissue. A visual scar (on the skin) you can readily see is composed of poorly developed skin, which has less resiliency than its surrounding tissues and will be more susceptible to breaking, in the event that it receives an abrasion. Inside the muscle the scar tissue is equally weak and possesses less mobility than surrounding muscles.

Body misalignment needn't be caused by a traumatic incident either; gravity is equally debilitating, but its influence is a very gradual one. Dr. Rolf considered gravity a major cause of the stresses on our bodies, as we daily fight the downward pull of gravity to remain upright. She held that gravity is what causes people to have poor posture and sagging muscles. It would be interesting to hear what the veteran U.S. astronauts have to say about weightlessness and its affect on body alignment.

Dr. Rolf reasoned that if you could get your body perfectly balanced, head balanced on top of the spine, spine balanced along its length and on top of the legs, legs straight and centered on the feet, then gravity could reinforce your balance. Getting that balance, though, isn't easy and requires loosening the fascia where it is stuck. This calls for applying pressure to the tissue in the direction it was originally intended to move. Since fascia is interconnecting, the entire body must be worked over.

If you've ever talked to someone who was rolfed you probably heard a story of pain, pleasure and a roller coaster of emotions, experienced during the ten one-hour sessions, which cost at least $40 per treatment. It's no picnic.

The rolf session begins with a series of photos of your body posture. The rolfer can see then just where you are out of alignment and where he needs to concentrate his work. Photos are taken before each session to track your progress.

A friend of mine went through the complete rolf treatment to see if it could help him with his chronic whiplash. He has had difficulty turning his head to the right ever since an auto accident severely twisted his neck out of alignment. His reaction to the treatment is typical of those who get rolfed. "Even though it was a ninety-minute session, it seemed to last only a few minutes. After the session I felt very spacey. Not stoned spacey, but very relaxed, ultra-serene. It's a difficult sensation to describe and unlike any I've ever experienced. My skin and muscles felt as if they were tingling." He said that he could, for the first time in a year, turn his head to the right without pain.

My friend said there were times, however, when he came home quite sore after a session. The first seven sessions concentrated on the individual parts of the body, such as chest, armpits (the most painful for him) legs, head and mouth. The last three sessions realign the entire body along its newly sculptured lines.

A kind of dependence developed for rolfing, my friend told me. "When I started getting rolfed, I'd go every other week and that was fine. But when I started to space out the appointments to once a month, I'd be tight and have the same knots in my neck and back by the time I saw the rolfer." And there is occasional pain, as my friend describes it: "Getting to the masseter muscle behind my jaw was not easy. The actual rolfing of the masseter and my gums was one of the most painful, unpleasant experiences of all the sessions. I was constantly gagging. After-ward, my mouth and gums ached for nearly two weeks."

Obviously, my friend had to have a certain dedication to see this treatment through the full ten sessions, but he says he defin-itely feels that it helped him and would recommend it to others. In the last three sessions, which are supposed to reintegrate the entire body along new lines, my friend said he experienced his best sensations. "After leaving each of those last three sessions, I felt ultra-loose, extremely confident, and tremendously decisive. I've retained at least some of those feelings." Also, the photos revealed a significant improvement in body alignment. "We ex-amined the Polaroids taken before and after every session. They were laid out on the table in sequential order; there was a notice-able (and dramatic) change in nearly every segment of my body. My head was no longer tilted to the left. I was nearly vertical and in alignment with my spine. My shoulders were broader and I was definitely standing straighter. I was less pigeon-toed and my knees were less turned in. I was taller by nearly a full inch."

Does rolfing work for everyone? Research on rolfing by Dr. Valerie Hunt, director of the Movement Behavior Laboratory at UCLA and Dr. Julian Silverman, a research specialist for the Cali-fornia Department of Hygiene, would indicate so. They held ex-periments at Agnews State Hospital in Santa Clara, California, in which subjects were tested before and after rolfing to learn if there were changes in neurological control of the muscles, for variations in response to stimuli and for biomechanical changes. Their find-ings supported what rolfers have been saying: There is more ef-ficient use of the muscles, conserved energy, increased refinement of response and a very real tendency for motor control to shift toward the spinal centers.

SHIATSU

Shiatsu means finger (shi) pressure (atsu) in Japanese, where the massage technique originated around the 18th century. Its basis is the recognition of a universal force, Chi, that flows through our bodies and must be kept free-flowing to maintain balance and health. Shiatsu serves to free up blocked passages, which are recog-nized by soreness, disease or injury. There are 365 acu-points throughout the body where the Shiatsu technician can apply the fleshy parts of his thumbs (the digit used most often), the palm of his hand or three fingers—index, middle and ring finger. The pressure lasts from five to seven seconds at any one pressure point.

Tokujiro Namikoshi, founder of the popular Nippon Shiatsu School, says that the basis of the science of Shiatsu is pure instinct and he gives this quotation, "The heart of shiatsu is like pure maternal affection. The pressure of the hands causes the springs of life to flow." Namikoshi, author of the book *Shiatsu,* points out that the technique cannot be successful if the person receiving the manipulations does not have the right mental attitude. He must believe in its force for it to succeed.

A more Western explanation for shiatsu and how it works is offered by Namikoshi. As we know, exhaustion is caused by an over-accumulation of lactic acid, a waste product of muscular contraction. Exhaustion can be relieved by suspending muscular action. By applying digital pressure over a muscle, says Namikoshi, it is possible to cause 80 percent of that acid to reconvert into glycogen. This eliminates fatigue more quickly and restores proper muscular balance. Shiatsu has its origins in acupuncture, an ancient Chinese treatment, commonly associated with needles.

Namikoshi is right when he says that you have to have the right frame of mind about a treatment. A friend of mine had shiatsu in San Francisco recently—her first time. She was used to the traditional full body massage using Swedish techniques and so she was not quite prepared for the shiatsu experience. "At times I found the manipulations painful and I wasn't expecting that," she said. "I don't know, maybe I wasn't in the right state of mind that day, because my friend, who also had the treatment, said she loved it and thought it was a great feeling." Which goes to show, you'll never know how you'll like it until you've tried it.

REFLEXOLOGY

Reflexology is an ancient therapy with roots from the Far East, and, once again, is an offshoot of acupuncture. Our organs and body parts have corresponding reflex points on other parts of the body, some of the most sensitive being those on the feet. The corresponding points are found by dividing the body into different zones. Organs lying in a particular zone can be stimulated by pressing various reflexes in the corresponding point zone. Working those tender reflexes helps rebalance the organs. From organ to reflex points are currents or pathways. Reflexology releases the blocks that don't allow the body energy to flow properly.

Although Western science does not yet have an explanation as to why reflexology works, some researchers are making inroads. Belgian chiropractor Dr. H. Gillet, in *Belgian Chiropractic Research Notes*, has found a correlation between the spine and feet. Acupuncture meridians, also used in reflexology, are still a mystery but Korean professor Kim Bong Han may have shed some light on their importance in the human anatomy. He has found a physical system (called *kyungrak*) of integrated ducts, which Dr. Han says are pathways for the meridians. These pathways are filled with fluid he calls *sanal*. Sanal contains DND, RNK and protein and is involved with cell formation.

Foot reflexology currently has the greatest following, although reflexology can be on other parts of the body, including the palms of the hands and even the ears (auriculotherapy). Devaki Berkson gives five reasons why the foot is so important in reflexology, in *The Foot Book:*

1) Strong energy poles of the body are linked to earth's energy emanations–sand, snow, grass, etc.

2) It's one of the most comfortable, non-threatening areas of the body to work.

3) Gravity and wear and tear accumulates large deposits of acids and tensions.

4) Foot reflexology soothes and deeply affects the person.

5) Foot reflex points are the most sensitive in the body.

The Chinese feel that the total body is reflected in the ear, eye, palm of the hand and bottom of the foot. They were the first to treat the feet with pressure; needles proved too painful. Dr. William H. Fitzgerald rediscovered this Chinese method of foot massage and brought it to the attention of the medical field in the United States in 1913, calling it "Zone Therapy." The technique consists of compression, using the thumbs to apply firm pressure. By doing compression over the entire foot, tender areas will indicate where concentration of treatment should be given. Twenty minutes is an adequate time to treat both feet. Pressure should be firm and not overly painful. During the treatment you are to lie down or prop yourself up in a chair, with your legs uncrossed. Crossing the legs blocks the free flow of energy.

You might perspire freely when getting a foot massage, according to Maybelle Segal, author of *Reflexology*. "Of course," she explains, "these reactions are caused because the body cannot accept the rapidity with which Nature gets rid of the toxins, and it reacts to this. If these reactions should occur while you are massaging, all you have to do is quickly massage the reflex area to the pituitary gland, which is the master gland." The vital organs should have their reflex zones massaged once a week—in acute cases, every third day. They should not be massaged more often, in order to give the organs the opportunity to recuperate from each removal of toxins.

Dr. Fitzgerald divided the body into ten zones vertically, five on the right and five on the left side. Tender areas indicate the body is not functioning properly and are caused by a deposit of crystalline waste products, which denote congested areas in the body. Foot massage will crush these deposits and then dissolve them, so that they can be carried away by the circulatory system.

REICHIAN MASSAGE

There probably isn't a massage form with a more bizarre history, entangling Albert Einstein, Sigmund Freud, the Food and Drug Administration and a box that supposedly could cure cancer. You might call Reichian massage a form of physical psychotherapy. In the right situation and with the right psychotherapist it can be quite effective in releasing pent-up frustrations and relaxing tense portions of the body.

The purpose of this massage is to assist physically, during counseling, in dissolving what Dr. Wilhelm Reich called "character armor." Reich believed that people subconsciously maintain muscular constriction in the torso, neck and head as a barrier against repressed emotions. He freed his patients of these repressed emotions by physically working on these tense areas during the usual verbal give-and-take associated with sessions on the couch.

The amount and type of massage you receive will vary considerably. It might last a couple of hours or much less, depending on how successfully your therapist breaks down the deep inhibitions. Also, it can be painful, with sharp jabs or pokes designed to stimulate certain reflexes, or lighter forms of stroking. Obviously, Reichian massage is recommended only for those who are also having emotional problems and should only be done by a trained therapist.

Dr. Reich broke the body into seven armor segments. His systematic breakdown won some support from psychoanalytic groups and furthered what would become an accepted form of therapy today. Treatment begins with the head and face, or what he called the ocular and oral rings. One technique frequently used to help dissolve ocular armoring is to get the patient to open his eyes repeatedly, as wide as he can. The deep neck musculature composed the third segment of armoring; a gag reflex is encouraged for releasing emotions here. The chest is the fourth segment, where armoring is marked by shallow breathing, and an area that Reich considered crucial in his treatment method. Reich identified a diaphragmatic segment as the fifth zone and the back muscles as the sixth segment. The seventh segment is the pelvis and the most crucial because it must ultimately be freed so that the individual's full orgasmic potential can be reached.

Dr. Reich considered the orgasm the crux of his controversial, albeit intriguing, theory of life. He believed that the universe is permeated by a primal, mass-free phenomenon that he called orgone energy. In the human organism the lack of repeated total discharge of this energy through natural sexual release is believed to be the reason for all neuroses and also the cause of "emotional plagues," irrational social movements and collective neurotic disorders.

Until Dr. Reich began taking his claims of orgone energy to the public, he was a respected staff associate at Sigmund Freud's Psychoanalytic Polyclinic in Vienna, Austria. After breaking with the institute he found his way to Norway after the Nazis forced him to leave Germany, and then to New York.

Reich's often distant and sometimes caustic personality would hinder his relations among fellow colleagues and with the public. He banked heavily on proving his theory of a life energy to Albert Einstein, whose support he believed would lend credibility to orgone energy. They met in Princeton, New Jersey in 1941 and at first Einstein agreed that further study of orgone energy was needed. However, he changed his mind soon after their meeting and thereafter would have nothing to do with Reich. Einstein's rejection of Reich came as a blow and marked the beginning of a series of events that would ruin Reich's already tarnished reputation.

Reich began marketing a plywood device he called the "orgone box," which he claimed would restore energy and supposedly could cure cancer. It was declared a fraud by the Food and Drug Administration and in 1956 he was tried for violation of the Food and Drug Act and sentenced to two years in a federal penitentiary, where he died one day before his release.

In the last decade, Reich's theory of a life force has generated renewed interest; TV personality Orson Bean wrote a book on his favorable experiences with psychiatric orgone therapy and scientists are beginning to take a closer look at this universal energy that captivated Dr. Reich and eventually proved his undoing.

JAMES CYRIAX

James Cyriax is a British physician who uses deep friction massage, which is popular with athletic trainers and many physical therapists, for the treatment of muscular, ligamentous and tendinous lesions. The massage technique is strictly therapeutic and can be painful, as it is designed to work deep muscle tissues that have been traumatized.

Deep friction does two things—includes traumatic hypermia and movement. Hypermia is the enhancement of the blood supply—similar to using heat but longer lasting. In the treatment of ligament damage Cyriax uses friction to disperse blood clots or effusion and moves the ligament over the subjacent bone to maintain its mobility. A day or two after a sprain, Cyriax recommends only light friction and very little movement, because there are no adhesions to break down at this point. For tendinous lesions, Cyriax rolls the tendon sheath back and forth against the tendon to smooth the gliding surfaces and to break up scar tissue.

Crucial to Cyriax' massage is transverse friction, as opposed to longitudinal friction, which merely moves blood and lymph along. Transverse friction moves the tissue itself. A stretching program is not always successful in loosening scar tissue, Cyriax says, because a stretched muscle's fibers lie more closely together, thus preventing the fibers from fully loosening.

TRAGER

Trager is not massage, although the goal of this bodywork is relaxation, the aim of both experiences. Nor is it concerned with muscle manipulation, although muscles are used as a medium. Rather, Trager Psychophysical Integration is, as the name implies, a method whose purpose is to reach the inner, subconscious mind to trigger relaxation. Dr. Milton Trager, a retired physician educated in Mexico and now living in Hawaii, stumbled onto his unique technique some fifty years ago, at the age of eighteen.

A casual observer watching a Trager session would see the practitioner shaking and vibrating the client's muscles and rocking and rolling the body. The movements are subtle, pain-free and require training to master.

Dr. Trager says he uses this particular approach because it is non-intrusive re-education that influences the release of deep-seated physical and mental patterns of limitation. These patterns can build up from the tensions of day-to-day living in a modern, highly mechanistic world. Or they may be the result of some traumatic injury, such as a fall. For example, you jam your shoulder and months later your muscles are still held in a protective mode. The shoulder lacks mobility and recurring muscle spasms are a problem. Instead of prying the muscle loose with deep massage, possibly a painful experience in itself, Trager Approach frees the locked muscle through gentle movements, which are designed to reach the mind so it can release the old holding patterns. Betty Fuller, director of the Trager Institute in Mill Valley, California, sees it this way: "I'm not trying to work on your physical body, but the physical body is like a telegraph key and the message I want to get through is to the autonomic nervous system, the one that runs the blood pressure, blood chemistry, body temperature and other functions we cannot consciously control. It will respond, bringing about release, relaxation and better function. Once experienced, the relaxed, peaceful feelings can be recalled consciously—thus bringing about the further release."

The practitioners are trained to work in a relaxed, meditative state of consciousness, which Dr. Trager calls "Hook-up." This state allows the practitioner to work effectively without fatigue and to become more sensitive to the patient's needs. There are no oils or powders used during the session, nor is it necessary to disrobe completely.

I wanted to know more about Trager and to experience it first-hand, so I called Betty Fuller at the Institute, a non-profit, tax exempt, public benefit corporation. Trager has become increasingly popular in the past decade and Dr. Trager has been able to devote full time to teaching and lecturing about his technique since retiring from his medical practice in 1977.

Betty said that not only did she want to discuss Trager with me, but that she would show me exactly what the experience feels like. My home in Mountain View was a convenient stop-off on the way to Esalen, where she would conduct a week-long training session, so she offered to pay a visit.

I was becoming more interested in learning different methods of relaxation and massage (besides writing a book on the subject) because of a recent accident that left me with a broken arm and knee-cap, as well as whiplash. I am like so many other injury victims—looking for some miracle cure for my aches and pains.

Betty arrived Sunday afternoon right in the middle of a key football game between the San Francisco 49ers and the Los Angeles Rams. If the 49ers won they were almost assured a division championship. This shouldn't have meant anything to Betty and me but I live in an apartment complex and a few units away there were some rabid fans cheering every great play the 49ers made. It wasn't exactly the atmosphere you look for when you're trying to relax. Betty made the best of the situation and suggested I turn on my TV so we could follow the game.

We had hardly introduced ourselves before I showed her a long, nasty-looking scar on my right arm. She grasped my arm with both hands, between my elbow and hand, and began shaking it gently, rhythmically. She had closed her eyes and appeared to be concentrating. "You might want to close yours, too, and relax," she suggested. My immediate reaction to her movements was favorable. Naturally, I tried to compare it to a sensation I had experienced previously, but was unsuccessful; this was something totally new. It was similar to vibration, but not exactly. My arm felt as though it had turned to a semi-solid state and it was waving back and forth. Betty moved up and down the length of my arm, pulled it away from and then pushed it back toward my side. "Now this is what I do, except over your entire body and with you lying down on a table. Does your arm feel more relaxed?" It did seem slightly more flexible, although I had managed to regain almost total mobility after several months of stretching. My strongest impression, however, came from the sensation of the arm moving so gently. I found it more relaxing than a massage.

I asked her about Mentastics, which is a part of the Trager Approach. She started shaking her hands and arms lightly, the way competitive swimmers shake them just before their race starts. "Mentastics are little movements that you do for yourself to enhance the feelings of lightness and freedom. The practitioner doesn't do them for you. Once you get the feeling of being light, you do it," Betty added. Her hands and arms fluttered about, as gracefully as butterfly wings. Dr. Trager developed this system of simple dance-like movements to maintain and enhance the sense of lightness, freedom and flexibility you gain from a Trager session. These playful movements are "mindfulness in motion," according to Dr. Trager, and can be effective in releasing accumulated stress. I lay down on my back next so that Betty could use Trager on my neck, as she stood behind me. Gently, she rocked my head back and forth. I was not encouraged to turn my neck, but to let it fall to the side. I had already been through five sessions of physical therapy, which included deep massage and joint manipulation, much of it quite painful. Tremendous progress had been made; however, my neck was still sore and stiff, especially when I turned it to the left. "There's no pulling, pounding or twisting here," she emphasized. "I don't do any cracking. I'm not going to suddenly get you loosened up and then snap anything. If anything makes you uncomfortable I want you to tell me." I felt no discomfort, as Betty promised. Occasionally she would stretch my neck by pulling on it gently with both hands. Betty reminded me not to stress the muscles in the neck. "I just want you to get the feel of being able to move your neck without pain."

She proceeded to show me more ways to move my neck and how to get up without using the neck muscles. Many of the movements Betty used on my neck I had experienced at The Massage Center in Palo Alto, California.

There was no rhythmic shaking of the neck. That aspect of Trager Approach seems to be most effective on the large muscles of the body, especially those on the arms and legs. While I did enjoy having my head rocked back and forth, it was not noticeably looser afterward, nor had I gained greater mobility. I had resigned myself to the realization, even before meeting Betty, that severe whiplash isn't something that will go away after a few treatments, whatever type they may be. It would take many more months before my neck was nearly back to normal. Strained ligaments and tendons respond slowly to treatment no matter what you do for them. Betty backed that up by saying that knees heal slowly, "There's just so much fibrous material, ligaments, tendons and bone."

During our discussion Betty told numerous stories of how Dr. Trager had successfully treated the severely crippled as well as improved the performance of athletes in a variety of sports using his method.

Because Betty was short on time, I did not experience a complete session of Trager, but she did have a chance to work on my legs. As I lay on my stomach she sat behind me and held one leg in the air by the foot. Her free hand conducted the same shaking action I received to the arm, only this time the sensation was even more relaxing. Any tightness I had was soon gone. This rocking technique can be applied to the entire body, as Betty showed me. She used just one hand, placed on my back, to rock my torso back and forth. In a search for words to describe the feelings I came up with: "primal." Her action had brought back fond childhood memories of being rocked to sleep.

Betty finished by stroking my back very lightly. She said that Trager uses a massage stroke on the back only, and added that it is not a massage motion designed to work the muscles; rather, it is a system that allows the client to appreciate the length of his back and its relation to the rest of the body.

Betty likes to emphasize the mental as well as physical side of Trager, and that it is not a medical treatment. She has written, "Psychophysical integration and mentastics is not in itself a medical treatment. If a medical doctor is doing it, of course, it is a medical treatment. It is actually a learning method; you are learning how your body can move . . . It is really a learning approach to using yourself well, to being a whole person, to having all your pieces and parts well integrated and coordinated."

If someone were to ask me what form of treatment is most effective at gaining complete relaxation, I would probably suggest Trager first, then massage. That is my biased opinion.

For more information on Trager and where you can find a certified Trager practitioner, write to Betty Fuller at The Trager Institute, 300 Poplar Avenue, Suite 5, Mill Valley, California 94941. Phone (415) 388-2688.

ACUPRESSURE (JIN-SHIN-DO)

You can't write about the ancient Chinese treatment of acupressure without tying in acupuncture. Their entire philosophy and execution are identical, with the important exception that acupressure does not include the use of needles; rather, the thumbs and fingers are used in their place. Acupressure is very much like shiatsu, but more strictly adheres to the meridians and energy pathways common to acupuncture.

Jin Shin Do and Jin Shin Jyutsu are Japanese versions of acupressure. Jin means compassion, Shin is spirit and Do is Tao, or way. Tao means the ultimate reality, everything that is. Jyutsu practitioners use their hands to press simultaneously at two different locations until an energy pulse is felt and then balanced. There is a sequence of fifty different movements for placing the hands.

The Chinese believe that there is a vital life force, called Chi (Ki in Japanese) that circulates through the human body along pathways or meridians, which follow a definite topographical pattern. So far, Western scientists have been unsuccessful at quantifying or registering Chi on instruments.

The Chi, which runs through the meridians, can be stimulated or blocked with the use of needles, or by the thumbs and fingers in the case of acupuncture. Along the meridians are thousands of sensitive points, called tsubos. They connect with the twelve main meridians. Two other meridians exist but they are different from the other twelve in that they do not constantly circulate energy.

Chi breaks down into two distinct forces, Yin and Yang. One does not exist without the other. When they are disproportionate in the body, that is always a sign of weakness or illness. Yin constitutes the following: feminine, darkness, night, passive, receptive, earth and moon, water. Yang is heaven or space, sky and sun, fire, light, day, active, assertive. The Chinese have gone further by breaking parts of the body down into areas of Yin and Yang. According to the Chinese theory of the universe, Yin and Yang produced the five elements—wood, fire, earth, metal and water—and from them all matter was fashioned. These elements are considered functions rather than inert substances.

Should you visit a skilled acupuncturist, he or she can diagnose your imbalances by monitoring your pulse. But this isn't the ordinary kind of pulse-taking you are familiar with, where the doctor counts for one minute. Meridians, those energy pathways, are located in the radial artery where the pulse is taken. An acupuncturist will take the pulse in both hands, simultaneously. Variations between the two pulses are used as a means of diagnosis. The right wrist is Yin and the left is Yang.

You are probably familiar with acupuncture needles, those long, silver slivers of steel (they can be gold or silver and vary in size) that insert into the skin. There should be no pain from an acupuncture needle that is inserted properly, during the insertion or afterward. Sometimes a patient will have dozens of needles sticking out of his body to the point that he looks like a porcupine, but will experience no pain. Acupuncture, in fact, is having its greatest impact on Western medicine in the field of anesthesia. An acupuncture needle placed in the right tsubo can deaden a large part of a body, so effectively that major surgery can take place without the use of other drugs, and the patient remains alert, talkative and pain-free.

Acupressure, of course, cannot do everything that the needles are capable of; it is primarily used to dislodge blocked meridians so as to allow the free flow of Chi. The procedure and affect is much like that of shiatsu.

POLARITY

Dr. Randolph Stone is responsible for establishing this form of treatment in the mid-1900s, after spending many years in India studying yoga and Eastern spiritual philosophies. The purpose of polarity is to bring the body into alignment through improved posture. The therapy is similar to rolfing, with heavy, concentrated pressure by the hands, thumbs or elbows. Dr. Stone describes patterns or lines of forces that operate throughout the body, similar to acupuncture, and that are closely associated with patterns of growth of the human fetus in the womb. He sees the body as having a plus and minus pole, just like a magnetic field, and by stimulating reflex points in terms of these poles, negative blockages can be neutralized, thereby establishing balance in the body.

ASTON-PATTERNING

This bodywork system, developed by Judith Aston, is similar to the Trager philosophy of releasing "holding patterns" in the body to guide the individual toward a more balanced and responsive way of living. Holding patterns can be physical in origin, caused by joint problems or our struggle to adapt to gravity. They can also be caused by inefficient ways of moving, sitting, sleeping and so on.

A major part of reducing these holding patterns through Aston-Patterning involves Neuro-Kinetics, which is a teaching system for understanding and experiencing ways to move the body more efficiently. The teacher guides you to an awareness of how you are using your body and how you can change to become more effective in your movements. You are encouraged to study your usual daily activities, rather than doing extraneous exercises or adopting postures your body is not ready to accept.

Additionally, there are two other systems the practitioner employs with Aston-Patterning; they are Arthro-kinetics and Myo-kinetics. Arthro-kinetics is a form of massage to work the joints, which helps to release holding patterns. Myo-kinetics does the same but with soft tissues.

Pain or discomfort is not part of Aston-Patterning and the average number of sessions a client goes through is from five to eight.

The director of the fitness lab at the S.M.A.R.T. health center in Cupertino, California, George Oehlsen, is just one of many who says he has benefited from Aston-Patterning. Oehlsen suffered severe whiplash in an auto accident and even after physical therapy and weightlifting he still had trouble moving his neck. He says that even though it was a year after the accident when he received Aston-Patterning, it gave him substantial new mobility in the neck.

TOUCH FOR HEALTH

Touch for Health is based on a combination of chiropractic and Oriental practices—such as shiatsu and acupuncture—used to improve muscle and postural balance. Many of the diagnostic and treatment methods are derived from applied kinesiology. Once muscle imbalances are identified, the practitioner can use any number of methods to restore structural balance, such as acupressure, lymphatic massage and so on. There is no set treatment.

Several years ago a chiropractor, at the National Running Week products show sponsored by *Runner's World* magazine, captivated his audience with his display of muscle manipulation. To the believer, he was doing nothing short of working miracles. But for the skeptics in the crowd, it was so much magic. Whatever your opinion, magic or miracle, this chiropractor was demonstrating one aspect of Touch for Health, a recent holistic health system, otherwise known as applied kinesiology, that continues to gain popularity.

Touch for Health defies categorization. It is neither massage nor bodywork. And yet it incorporates both systems into its makeup. Add a sprinkling of Far Eastern health beliefs, nutrition, holism and chiropractic and you have Touch for Health.

A group of American chiropractors is responsible for establishing the Touch for Health Foundation, which is the organizational body overseeing those who practice applied kinesiology on the professional level. In the early 1960s applied kinesiology was "discovered" by George Goodheart, a Detroit chiropractor. He found that tight muscles were not really caused by spasms, but that weak muscles on one side of the body would cause normal muscles, opposing the weak ones, to become tight. Another chiropractor, John Thie, of Pasadena, California, spearheaded the organization of the Foundation several years later, after studying Goodheart's ideas. He is the current president and author of *Touch for Health,* a landmark book published in 1973, which describes the technique of applied kinesiology. It is written for the lay person who wants to use muscle testing on family or friends.

Applied kinesiology has perhaps gained the most notoriety in sports medicine, in recent years, through the efforts of Pasadena, California, chiropractor Dr. Leroy Perry, Jr. Perry has had great success with athletes, most notably in track and field. Dwight Stones attributes his world-record high jump to Perry's skilled hands. Despite his huge success, Perry, because he is not a medical doctor, was barred from serving on the 1976 Olympic medical team, much to the disappointment of American athletes. However, in Montreal he represented the small island nation of Antigua and worked on dozens of athletes from around the world, including Untied States team members.

It is understandable why the traditional sports medicine establishment does not want applied kinesiology gaining a foothold when you consider that it emphasizes non-drug therapy. Touch for Health might just symbolize the epitomy of holistic medicine, the belief that body, mind and spirit must be treated as a "whole." Thie says that Touch for Health takes into account the physical, mental and spiritual aspects of being. "And the unique contribution of touch healing is that the lay person is provided with a therapeutic tool—it can be used by husband and wife, parent and child, or simply two friends, as a means of unblocking or balancing energy."

This energy, Thie says, is universal. "We are all one with the universe, with the universal energy. When this energy is highly concentrated, we call it "matter," and our bodies *are* that matter. Therefore, our bodies are literally this universal energy, in some of its various forms."

According to Thie, this energy has been understood by Far Eastern medicine for thousands of years. Their doctors have mapped it along what are called meridians, or energy pathways in the body. They are a key factor in understanding how Touch for Health works. Meridians are said to contain a free-flowing, noncellular liquid that the Chinese call chi. Along the meridians are some five hundred points—small oval cells that are electromagnetic in character. In China, acupuncture treatment and acupressure deal with these points. Thie believes that we are nurtured from the outside with energy and that the "energy-entering" points are the points of Chinese acupuncture. "They act like little antennas, and when we touch them in the healing process, it is as though we were acting as auxiliary antennas, as we do when we touch the antenna points on a radio or television, infusing them directly into energy."

To find out how well energy is flowing within the body and to isolate imbalances in this energy, muscle testing is used; it is what makes Touch for Health unique among all of the bodywork forms. It is a simple way of diagnosing your body. A muscle that tests weak indicates some blockage or constriction in the energy flow. The process of unblocking the energy and restoring balance is called balancing. Touch for Health is not a healing system or a cure-all. The practitioner merely acts as a medium to find weaknesses and then lets the body concentrate on healing that area.

To test a muscle, the body is placed in a certain position, which brings the ends of the muscle being tested closer together, and puts other muscles that ordinarily work with it at a disadvantage. The practitioner then presses in a direction that requires the muscle being tested to work to hold the body in position. If the muscle is weak, meaning that it is shaky, or allows the arm or leg to give way under the muscle test, it indicates that the flow of energy in that system needs to be stimulated. During testing, you remain fully clothed. There are no oils used. Generally, you are asked to lie down for the tests, although many tests can be done while standing.

A weak muscle can also indicate possible trouble with that muscle's related organ. Every group of muscles has a related organ.

There are various systems used to strengthen weak points. You can use any one or a combination of the following techniques.

● **Neuro-lymphatic massage**—Energy to the lymphatic system is regulated by the neuro-lymphatic reflexes, located mainly on the chest and back. These reflex points act like circuit breakers, which get turned off when the system is overloaded. The neuro-lymphatic points vary in size from that of a pellet to a small bean. They are usually tender. To work the neuro-lymphatic reflexes, a practitioner moves around the point for that particular muscle with his fingers, using a deep massage and applying pressure for twenty to thirty seconds.

● **Neuro-vascular holding points**—They are located mainly on the head. A practitioner holds them with the pads of his fingers for a few seconds. This appears to improve the blood circulation to both the muscle and related organ.

● **Meridians**—The flow of energy through a meridian may be stimulated by using the hands to trace the meridian line in the proper direction on the surface of the body. It is only necessary to come within two inches of the meridian, either off to the side or even above the skin and over clothing.

● **Acupressure holding points**—Those points on the same side of the body as the muscle that is weak are used. The first arm and leg points are held at the same time, one with each hand. The practitioner maintains light pressure for about thirty seconds.

● **Nutrition**—A muscle weakness may be caused by a nutritional deficiency normally associated with that particular muscle. A practitioner can give you a food containing a concentrated amount of the necessary nutrient. The body responds positively to the required nutrient by exhibiting a strong muscle during testing.

I first learned of Touch for Health from a friend, while researching the book. I decided to pursue the subject further and consulted the book *Healthsource*, a guide to massage and bodywork practitioners in the Bay Area. I was surprised to see the name of Helga Brandt; I know her two sons, but I didn't know about her profession. Helga works out of her home in Menlo Park, California, and is certified in Touch for Health, Swedish massage and is a professional tennis instructor.

After discussing Touch for Health and getting to know one another, at which time I told her about my accident, she pulled out her massage table and set it up.

For her to do muscle testing, all I had to do was lie down on the table on my back. Quickly and efficiently she went through the muscle tests. She started with my left arm, the one that was broken six months previous. I was asked to extend it out to my side and parallel with the floor. As she stood at my left side, she pulled it toward my body with one of her hands. I had no trouble resisting her effort. Over the past six months I had worked the muscle back almost to its old strength and flexibility. But after the first test she tried something different. She placed the fingertips of her right hand in the middle of my chest, on the thyamus gland. She re-tested the left arm. I was unable to resist her effort when she pulled down on my arm. Helga said that the thyamus gland is a good information source; it was indicating an imbalance in my anterior deltoid muscle.

Next she tested my right arm and found no imbalances. The same was true for my legs. Despite breaking a kneecap six months ago, I had re-built the atrophied muscles through bicycle riding. Throughout the testing I was asked to either resist or push against her force.

I knew I would show some muscle imbalance when she tested my neck, because I had been the victim of whiplash. I turned onto my stomach and she tested the neck muscles from there. That set of muscles was fine. Then I turned onto my back again for more testing. I was asked to lift my head off the massage table and tilt it to one side. From this position she took hold of my head with one hand and put her other hand on my shoulder. I was asked to resist the force of her hand as she pushed it toward my shoulder. The muscles were weak. "You have weak anterior neck muscles," she said.

Helga then ran her hands over my body, but never touched me. She looked like someone using a Ouija board. She left the room and went into the kitchen and returned holding something in her hand. She asked me to extend my left arm again. She placed the object

that was in her hand, a clear capsule, on my chest, over the thya-
mus gland. We went through the muscle testing routine once again.
This time my arm was strong! I was able to resist her efforts.
"What is that pill you put on my chest?" I asked.

"This is 25,000 units of vitamin A," she said.

I couldn't believe that. "Why vitamin A?" I asked, with some
doubt in my voice.

Helga said that, based on my type of muscle imbalance, she
knew my body was in need of that particular nutrient. I didn't believe it. "Let's try another kind of pill," I said firmly. I thought I
could trip her up if she used a different pill. I believed that any
pill would work.

She went back into the kitchen and came out with another pill.
We went through the arm test again. This time my arm was weak!
"Now what kind of pill is that?" I asked in disbelief.

"Vitamin C," she said.

I didn't know what to make of this. The left half of my mind,
the rational half, wanted further testing, while the right half was
ready and willing to believe everything that happened, no matter
how unscientific her testing might have been. Then it dawned on
me. I had only recently started buying carrots at the grocery store.
I hadn't bought carrots for over a year. I remember walking
through the fresh produce section and making a conscious decision
to buy the carrots. Maybe my body was trying to tell me something.

To prove her point, Helga returned to the kitchen and this time
came out with a carrot. "Now eat this," she said. I took a bite. We
retested my left arm. It was stronger, but not quite as strong as
when she used the vitamin A pill.

As a system of diagnosing muscle imbalances, applied kinesiology appears to be invaluable. That it can also serve as a tool for
recognizing nutritional deficiencies I found remarkable. While the
right half of the mind enjoyed the experience and I certainly
gained from it, the left half continues to question, as it rightly
should, the entire process. Now it wants me to try it again, only
this time using the double-blind experiment method. And if it
still works, then we'll try . . .

To find your nearest certified Touch for Health practitioner,
write Touch for Health, 1174 N. Lake Avenue, Pasadena, California 91104.

CHIROPRACTIC

Chiropractic, German for doing by hand, can be considered the grandfather of bodywork. This method of treatment was first introduced in the United States by D.D. Palmer in 1895 and carried on by his son, Bartlett Joshua Palmer. It has legal recognition in the United States, and there are numerous training institutions.

Chiropractic theory maintains that vertebral displacement causes pressure on the nerves that pass from the spinal cord to different parts of the body. Misalignment of the spine interferes with the transmission of nerve impulses, which contributes to disease and pain in movement.

There are various means of identifying the unaligned vertebrae, such as feeling the back and spine, taking x-rays, observing a person's manner of walk and through applied kinesiology.

Chiropractors are famous for cracking people's backs, a method called "adjustment." Massage is also an important part of therapy, because tight muscles protecting a misaligned vertebra can prevent adjustments from being effective.

While chiropractic can be a highly effective treatment for people with bad backs, the client should be sure that his chiropractor has been certified by one of the established institutions.

OSTEOPATHY

Dr. Rolf gained many of her theories about bodywork from osteopathy, which has been around for over a century. It is German for bone treating. This school of medicine was founded in 1874 by A.T. Still and concerns itself with the relationship of the musculoskeletal system to health and disease. It maintains that the normal body produces forces necessary to fight disease, but can break down with "structural derangement." This occurs with frequent slight strains, which eventually are capable of causing misalignment of bones and cartilage, all of which are termed "lesions."

In the United States, colleges of osteopathy are accredited by the American Osteopathic Association. Osteopaths emphasize drugless health care, although it is legal for them to prescribe drugs and practice surgery.

FELDENKRAIS METHOD

Feldenkrais is a bodywork system involving exercises that the client does and body movements executed by the practitioner, as systematized by Moshe Feldenkrais. Feldenkrais, 77, born in Russia and now living in Israel, became interested in the way the body functions when, in 1940, a Glasgow surgeon told him that he needed an operation for his bad knee and that it had only a fifty-fifty chance of success. Although his expertise was in physics (he has a doctorate from the Sorbonne) and mechanical engineering, Feldenkrais decided that he would begin a study of the mechanics of body movement to see if he could cure his knee.

In 1947, his research culminated in the publication of *Body and Mature Behavior: A Study of Anxiety, Sex, Gravitational and Learning*, his first of three books. Twenty years later, the holistic health movement brought him to North America, where his work elevated him from the status of obscurity to mind-body guru. During the formative years in Israel, where he received support from David Ben-Gurion, who Feldenkrais brought back to health, his system was perfected.

Feldenkrais is especially interested in how man learns and in his ability to develop new responses to stimuli. He says that any function involving voluntary muscle activity must pass through a period of apprenticeship, at which time the neural pathways are formed. Neural activity tends to follow pathways already traveled and this probability increases through repetition. For example, if you strain a calf muscle and begin to limp, even after the healing you will probably continue limping, because of the re-education that has gone on in the neural pathways.

The limits imposed on the range of movement are not found in the muscles, but at a higher level of organization of the nervous system. A neural reorganization in the cortex is necessary to change patterns of behavior, one of Feldenkrais's favorite beliefs. The motor cortex has many connections and nerve cells that are directly related to specific muscles that produce specific movements. If the muscle patterns are never altered, then those regions of the brain remain in fixed patterns. Feldenkrais says that if you utilize as many of your muscular aparatus as possible, the more aware you are of those movements the more the brain will be activated. The more parts of the brain that function well, the better the whole brain will work.

Feldenkrais manipulates the client's muscles to introduce correct learning patterns, but Professor Karl Pribram, head of the Neuropsychology Labs at Stanford University, says it is more than just muscle work that Feldenkrais uses, "He's not just pushing muscles around. He's changing things in the brain itself so that the patient can gradually adjust his whole muscular dysfunction to what we call a normal image. In the motor cortex there's a photographic image which I call an image of achievement. And it's that whole image which Feldenkrais transmits."

Functional Integration, part of the Feldenkrais Method, is conducted on a one-to-one basis with the practitioner and involves the body manipulation aspect of Feldenkrais. Awareness Through Movement, the other half of Feldenkrais, is usually carried out through group workshops and consists of gentle stretching exercises lasting about one hour, which are designed to teach the body proper movement.

Functional Integration takes place with the client lying prone, to facilitate the breaking down of habitual muscular patterns. The lessons are done slowly, with no pain or strain and the objective is to discover unknown new reactions in oneself and thereby learn a better, more congenial way of acting. Lightness of movements is a major concern, Feldenkrais says. This produces the maximum sensitivity in the person.

Feldenkrais has conducted numerous workshops around the country, where Feldenkrais practitioners receive their training. Of sixty-six Americans who enrolled in his first American training, sixty-three stayed the entire three years.

For more information about Feldenkrais practitioners, contact The Feldenkrais Guild, 1776 Union St., San Francisco, California 94123.

CANINE MASSAGE

Yes, animals love to be massaged, too. The Society for the Prevention of Cruelty to Animals will just love you for treating your pet to a full body massage, and your pet will love you, too. If you're really serious about giving your pedigree show dog the full treatment, I doubt that any practitioner will do you the favor, but there is an alternative—do it yourself with help from *The Art of Canine Massage*, a large-format paperback complete with photos demonstrating different strokes. There's even a chart showing a dog's paw, for those interested in canine reflexology. Ursula Major wrote it and you can own it by writing to Bjornhardt Publications, 3285 S. Court, Palo Alto, California 94306.

3

Life at a Massage Center

Perhaps no other people in the United States have a greater interest in, more access to or heightened awareness of massage than the residents of the San Francisco Bay Area. This is the Mecca for those who seek further insights into their place in society, into the way they live, into a holistic orientation to life. Hundreds of human growth centers have sprung up here since the heady, drug-expressive days of the 1960s. From Mill Valley in the north, to Berkeley in the east and south to San Jose, they offer a variety of services—yoga, massage, psychotherapy, group counseling and so on. They are staffed by some of the most innovative and experienced professionals in the country.

The Massage Center in Palo Alto is one such establishment, recently celebrating its tenth anniversary. Palo Alto is one of a dozen or so suburb communities that occupy a narrow peninsula extending from San Francisco to San Jose. Palo Alto marks the northern boundary of what is now called Silicon Valley, the heart of our country's computer industry.

The success of The Massage Center, besides the quality of service always offered there, is due in part to the unique social and health awareness that Palo Alto residents share. Stanford University, the "Harvard of the West," is nearby. Stanford Hospital takes up part of the sprawling campus and is the site of some of the world's most advanced medical breakthroughs; recently, surgeons there performed the first successful heart-and-lung transplant on a human. But the readily available and advanced medical practices in Palo Alto share equal footing with numerous holistic-minded facilities, such as the San Andreas Health Council and Midpeninsula Health Center. The existence of this new-wave health orientation that stresses preventive medicine is clearly an expression of the needs and desires of the people of Palo Alto. They are healthy, sensitive and liberal-minded, people who want the most out of life in a land that has so much to offer. They are cyclists, equestrians, runners, skiers, sailors . . . Two of the best-known bicycle shops in the country, Palo Alto Bicycles and Wheelsmith, are right downtown. The city provides for its residents a unique, free door-to-door trash recycling pick-up service. Linus Pauling, Nobel Prize winner and the man who gave vitamin C its notoriety, has an office overlooking the city.

Two blocks off University Avenue, the heart of Palo Alto, is The Massage Center, on Bryant, a quiet, residential street. The center shares a modest one-story, wood-frame building with several other businesses and has been at this location since its inception. Unlike most massage centers, this is a cooperative business and it presently has eight staff members. They share equally in the financial rewards, and the responsibilities of running the business. Some are long-time Palo Alto residents, while others have found their way here from all corners of the country. They are young, energetic and dedicated.

A few of you who read this book have had a massage before, but most of you have not. You may not have a massage center nearby. The recent wave of interest in holistic health—which includes massage—has still not reached many areas of the country, partly because of conservative attitudes and partly because the demand just might not be there. You may live in a small community where not many people are interested in a sensual, revitalizing, humanistic massage—or even know that there is such a thing. If you mention massage to them they may think you're talking about an activity that occurs in the red-light district of the nearest big city. A certain percentage of you are willing and ready to receive a non-sexual massage but you are just a little hesitant about the whole experience. You have some questions or misunderstandings about the step-by-step process of what goes on. You might wonder what the people who give massage are like. Are they different? Do they have magic powers? Just why are they in this line of work, anyway? You might wonder how a massage center operates. We are often afraid to get involved in something we know nothing about. We like the security of knowing exactly what will transpire in whatever endeavor we undertake, and that especially applies to being a client in a therapist/client relationship. How does a massage center operate? How much does a massage cost and what types of massage are available?

The following interviews will go a long way toward answering your questions and reducing your worries about having that first massage, that first sensual experience. Two long-time members of The Massage Center, Marcia Nelson (since 1977) and Michael Murphy (since 1972), give details on how their center works and offer personal insights into the practitioner's side of the business.

Q. Could you give a brief history of The Massage Center? Who were its first patrons?

A. The founders were a group of people who had either recently finished training in massage or who had been working in massage at some other place. The person who was the prime mover was Donna Gerry. She had strong feelings about working in a place that supported the idea of massage as a healthful, beneficial and therapeutic enterprise.

She had worked in massage studios and found that the atmosphere was generally unsupportive of the therapeutic, holistic work she was doing. She wanted a place where the whole environment suggested a reputable, therapeutic, relaxing experience.

Donna realized that the only way she could have the right atmosphere was to start her own place. She chose a collective partnership rather than an employer/employee structure, and The Massage Center was founded in 1971.

Donna and five others started the business in its present location on Bryant Street. They barely had enough money to pay the first and last month's rent. At that point she had no more funds to paint it or furnish it. But everyone chipped in. There were some rough times at the beginning but after the first eighteen months they were open they had paid off all the initial loans. They were making about thirty-three cents on the dollar back then, so that if the practitioner did an hour's massage she would get a third of what the massage client paid the center. Not much.

Q. How is the business structured? How does your cooperative work?

A. We are eight partners with equal ownership and decision-making power in the business. A client will call us or come into the Center and say "I'd like a massage from Linda, or Michael, or Marcia." Or, "I'd like to have a massage on Tuesday afternoon. Who's available then?"

Q. Prices?

A. Right now (March 1982) it's $20 for a half hour, $30 for an hour and $40 for an hour-and-a-half massage.

Q. What permits are required of your business?

A. There are two. One is a use permit that says we're going to use the establishment as a commercial business. The other permit is one that allows us to be operating what is called an "adult entertainment enterprise." The city still sees massage in the category with adult books and peep shows. So, although they know that we're a straight establishment, they still have an ordinance that restricts us along with all of the other kinds of massage places.

Q. Do the police check your business?

A. When the ordinance first went into effect they inspected all the places in town. We assume that we were checked at that time but we were never made aware of it. Occasionally we had a client who seemed a little "suspicious," and we wondered if that was what was going on.

Q. How do you advertise The Massage Center?

A. We advertise in the daily newspaper, a weekly newspaper and *Common Ground*, which is a newsprint magazine that lists various practitioners, massage, bodywork, and so on, in the Bay Area. And the telephone book. Most of our clients find out by word of mouth. We also have a brochure and occasionally we will use postering.

Q. Do you offer instructional classes?

A. Yes. Most of our massage classes are taught by The Massage Center partners, although occasionally we will have a guest instructor. We offer three categories of classes:

1. **Weekend workshops.** They are short classes, usually held on Saturdays for three to six hours. These are ideal for people who simply want an introduction to massage and just want to learn the basics of how to give an enjoyable massage to family and friends, or who want to brush up on techniques they have already acquired.

Workshops cover a variety of subjects, including Introduction to Massage; Back, Neck and Shoulder Massage; Head, Hands and Feet Massage; Acupressure; Breathwork and Massage; Parent-Child Massage; Special Problems for Massage Therapists, and so on.

2. **Series classes.** They meet one night a week for six to ten weeks and offer the massage enthusiast a chance to more thoroughly learn techniques for giving an effective, relaxing and nurturing massage. Class subjects include Beginning and Intermediate Massage; Anatomy and Advanced Massage; How Bodies Work; Acupressure; Massage and Healing, and so on.

3. **The Massage Certification Course.** This is a 200-hour training program for individuals who want comprehensive, in-depth instruction to prepare them to do professional-quality massage. Most of these students plan to earn part or all of their living as massage practitioners, yet many people take this course as a way of furthering their own personal growth.

Our Certification Course is longer and more thorough in its training than most other massage schools. The State Department of Private Postsecondary Education approves all massage schools and sets minimum curriculum guidelines that all schools must meet. Many schools limit their curriculum to these minimum guidelines set by the state, and we have often been disappointed in the lack of quality of the massage that has resulted. Since we want and expect our graduates to excel as practitioners, naturally our coursework reflects our high standards and is very comprehensive.

Q. Does a massage student take a final test of some kind?

A. We require a practical exam at the end of the course. When a student has satisfactorily completed all of the coursework, he or she must massage one of the instructors. If the massage is of professional quality, the student passes and is certified.

Q. In what ways does The Massage Center work to separate its image from that of a sex-oriented massage parlor?

A. Liberal use of the word "therapeutic" in our advertising. We mention that we offer our services to women. Whenever we get a phone call from a man that we know hasn't been by here we tell him outright that we don't offer any sexual services. We really pound it in. Plus, we have no red carpeting on the floor, no dark rooms (laughter). We also avoid any words or phrases that might be interpreted as meaning sexual massage.

Q. What do you think has been the key to the success of The Massage Center?

A. We give a very good massage. Our standards are very high. It's hard to get a job at The Massage Center. We demand a knowledge and skill that is well above average. We never take a student right out of class. Usually people have been certified for a year or more.

Also, people's attitudes are changing, and that has helped enormously. In the early days of The Massage Center, most of our clients were people who had been exposed to massage through the Midpeninsula Free University, or people who had experienced massage at Esalen, or even those who had experienced it in Europe and knew of its therapeutic value. These clients would come to get help in relaxing tight muscles, or to improve circulation, or to increase flexibility. Slowly but surely, more people would learn about massage as an adjunct to personal growth or as something that can be valuable in relationship to physical fitness and personal stress control. People are understanding massage to be a valid and important aspect of their health care. Not only do people think of massage as something that feels good, they find that massage, because of its ability to help a person relax, assists them in coping, physically and emotionally, in their everyday lives. And part of the reason that people's attitudes are changing is that more and more people are receiving massage. They tell their friends and more people become comfortable with the idea of massage as an acceptable thing to do.

Q. What types of massage does The Massage Center offer? Bodywork?

A. Our massage is a combination of Esalen and Swedish styles. It is slower than Swedish and deeper than Esalen. If people ask for Jin Shin Acupressure, Shiatsu, Applied Kinesiology, Trager, Rolfing, or some other specialty, we will refer them to the person in the cooperative who specializes in that particular approach.

Q. How did you become practitioners?

A. (Marcia) I was a biofeedback technician for a year and a half where I worked for a psychiatrist. I liked it, but I felt limited by having to work with the equipment. I wanted a type of contact that was more personal, more creative. I took classes in massage and found that I liked it. I became certified, then began working at The Massage Center in 1977.
(Michael) I was an undergraduate student of psychology and active in a project that was designed to make psychology less abstract and theoretical. We ran encounter groups, tours of mental hospitals, bioenergetics workshops and other programs to make psychology more personally relevant to the students. A group of us within the project was especially interested in body-oriented subjects. We had a Rolfer come and talk to us. We took massage classes and some yoga. Massage quickly became something that I did well. Friends would come to me and ask for help with their physical pains and tensions. I studied on my own for several years and then, in 1972, I moved to Palo Alto, where I met several people at The Massage Center. They invited me to come by and

hang out and I'm still hanging out nine years later.

(Marcia) My family is medically oriented. My mother was a nurse and my father is a doctor. I always had that focus—of being interested in health care, in very traditional ways. When I discovered the holistic health spectrum, specifically massage and acupressure, that interested me more. It took a while before my family accepted what I was doing. They understood that I was doing legitimate massage but they weren't comfortable with the idea; they had no context for it. Then my mother heard a program on the radio talking about massage as being helpful for stress reduction, and a positive reference was made to The Massage Center in Palo Alto. That suddenly made what I was doing acceptable to my parents. Now they send me newspaper clippings about massage and acupressure; they've become very supportive.

Q. How do you get used to the idea of touching someone as a way of doing a job?

A. (Marcia) There's a depersonalization going on when I touch someone at work. It is close and personal, but clinical as well. It is personal in the sense that I am relating to your muscles, your skin, where it's tense, where it's loose and so on. But it's a client-therapist relationship.

(Michael) The intimacy of a massage is much different than what we normally feel in, say, a friendship. In a friendship, the relationship is a two-way relationship, but as your masseur, I'm there for you. My feelings, my emotions, my moods are more in the background. The service of the massage is most important.

Q. How do you deal with your moods during the massage?

A. (Marcia) There's a switch that flips when I go in to do a massage. Whatever else that is going on drops into the background. I focus on the person I'm working with.

(Michael) Friends ask me what I do when I'm feeling very sad and I'm crying. I tell them that I make sure I don't get my tears on the client (laughter). It's part of the way that works best for me, not to hold in all my emotions. I have to find a way of letting them out, but at work I don't dwell on them with my clients.

Q. What's the most enjoyable aspect of your job? The least enjoyable?

A. (Michael) The best part is being with somebody and assisting them in letting go of something bad, something that has been a real strain on them. There's something about being part of that release. It's really exhilarating. It's inspiring. If that person can let go of that much pain and tension and tightness then there's hope for all of us.

(Marcia) For me it involves shifting to a different state of awareness, a different perspective. When you meditate, for example, your focus is on a different level. It's not an everyday-relating kind of level that most of us live in. Massage brings my awareness to a different phase, similar to meditation. Someone can come in and be very guarded, and talking between us may be a little bit awkward. Maybe they're a little nervous and don't know what to expect. They lay on the table and I start working. I'm relating to them on different levels. I'm still relating to their personality. I'm also relating to their body—noticing and working with their physical tensions, watching relaxation take place, feeling tension dissolve under my fingertips. Emotional holding is also a part of physical tension. So, as muscles relax there is an accompanying emotional letting go. Sometimes the emotional release takes the form of crying, or sighing, or maybe a new sensation of joy. Whatever the client's particular experience, there is usually a noticeable relief from physical and emotional stress, along with an increased sense of well-being. I can feel the change as I witness it. That is satisfying.

Teaching is also a great experience. It comes from teaching people new things. In massage, people learn to sense more on an energy level, more on an intuitive level. They're constantly making very personal discoveries for themselves that they may not have ordinarily thought of as being part of massage. When people take a class, very often they're just thinking about how to physically manipulate muscles so it will feel good and so the other person can relax. Yet there's a whole aspect of massage that is more on an energy level, more sensing. Parts of them begin to unfold when they're doing massage, parts that they don't think of at other times—different ways of relating to the person on the table and different ways of viewing the whole world. Sometimes the whole class will get that; they'll just make a shift to a different level. They're not trying to. It's just being presented as part of the material and suddenly they get it.

(Michael) When people come to a massage center to learn a technique, they think they're going to learn a skill. What they really find out they're learning is maybe a new way of relating to themselves and to the other people in the class. So they carry that personal skill into their bodywork, as well as how to use their hands. There's more to this all of a sudden.

(Marcia) I'm teaching a beginning massage class now and so far we've been focusing on how to do the strokes. This week we had a class and didn't use massage strokes. All we did was energy work.

The students felt how very effective they were without really "doing" anything except experiencing the power of conscious touch. These students experienced the effectiveness of sensing energy and consciously directing it, whether they were massaging or simply touching. What it means is that their massage work has gone to a new level.

(Michael) It also helps if you have an artistic sense and you find it easy being with people.

Q. Negative aspects?

A. (Marcia) Sometimes people are very resistant. They want me to make them feel totally relaxed and they don't want to let go of anything in the process. They totally turn the job over to me.They want me to make them feel better but they just don't want to change. On the other hand, some people try too hard to relax, but for them the experience is often still so new. They need to have a couple more massages. After a while their bodies learn how to relax and how to let go of trying.

(Michael) Of course, then there are people who bounce checks with us or don't pay their bill. That's the unpleasant side of the business.

Q. Can you describe a good massage experience?

A. (Marcia) A good example of one occurred on Monday. I was

massaging a woman in her late-sixties. I could tell that her muscles were really letting go and relaxing. It was a really nice experience to massage her. When I asked her to turn over she said, "Now don't laugh at me, but this feels like a religious experience." I didn't laugh. I said, "I know what you mean, because some people have that experience."

Then, when I was massaging her face and her head, tears just started streaming down her face. She didn't say anything about it. Nobody had to say anything. It was just like she was *really* being touched. I don't know what emotions she was feeling or what it was bringing up in her, but she was just feeling an opening in herself and a need was being fulfilled. It was a very, very personal experience for her that went deeper than what you might think of as just going in and just having your muscles relaxed and massaged. That illustrates what I mean about massage touching people on different levels. Some people often get more out of massage than they intend to. It just brings people more in touch with themselves. At the same time that brings me more in touch with those levels of myself and of other people because I'm right there being part of the experience.

(Michael) I'm constantly aware of the fact that my work brings me in touch with people who are, in main, willing to let go down to those levels. It's inspiring.

Q. Isn't it uncommon for someone to cry during a massage?

A. (Marcia) I would say that at least 50 percent of the people who get massaged feel some amount of what that woman was experiencing. Most people don't express it as fully as she did. Most people don't cry. Probably at least 5 percent of those massaged do cry and express themselves outwardly. I've told this experience to a few friends and they said, "Yep, I know exactly what that woman meant."

Q. How about income in your profession. Is it lucrative?

A. (Michael) No.
(Marcia) My limitation is that I can't do forty massages a week. I can't even do twenty. Even though we charge $30 an hour, you can't do enough massages to get rich. But obviously you can make a living. We do. For most people it's a part-time job.

Q. That leads to the next question. How many massages do you do every day?

A. (Michael) Well, I did eight on Monday. Today I did six.
(Marcia) I feel comfortable doing only two or three a day. I used to do about sixteen a week. Now I like to do eight or less a week. I find that after doing about twelve to sixteen a week for three years I just don't want to do so many anymore. I need to do other types of work, too, like administrative work, teaching, phone work and so on.

Q. Do you find that you need to get psyched up for the massage?

A. (Marcia) Not usually. Sometimes if I'm just really tired or dragged out a change takes place when I go to work. Once I get in there and put on the oil and talk to the person, a shift takes place. I'm present and I'm ready to massage.
(Michael) I notice that at the end of the day, the last session usually feels fine. Then I go, "Okay, that's the last session." If, an hour later, somebody wants another session, I've already unplugged for the day. If I had planned to do another massage then I could have kept going. But after I've unhooked and started to unwind for the day it's hard to get back up for a massage.

Q. Can you describe how your work attitude has changed since giving your first professional massage?

A. (Marcia) I've gotten a lot less defensive about giving a massage. In the beginning I sometimes had trouble massaging men who didn't seem to understand all the various levels we have been talking about, concerning massage. I was always on the defensive that they were really going to be wanting a sexual massage. Occasionally I was right and a lot of times I was wrong. But just as society associates massage with a sexual experience, I was afraid that the men would keep making that association. It took me a while to be comfortable about the whole issue.

I love it a lot more now. I feel like I've really been able to grow in terms of doing massage. I've become more creative in doing massage and can tap in more easily on various levels with whomever I'm working with and that makes it more rewarding for me. I feel more effective and present in my work.

(Michael) The more experienced I become and the more I know about what's possible, the better I am able to take massages to the limits of what's possible than I was in the beginning. At first I would do a massage and nice things would happen almost by accident. Now I've begun to understand some of the parameters that help to make a massage a really profound experience for somebody. So my work is more consistently at a profound level now than it was before.

Q. Can you recount your first experience giving a professional massage?

A. (Marcia) One of the first people I massaged was a woman who had had many massages. I was massaging away, hoping I was doing the right thing. She was lying face-up and I reached under her back to hold some acupressure points and she started crying. I forget what she was crying about, but I was so thrilled that I had done something right. She had appreciated the experience and was glad to be able to release some painful emotions she had been holding back from herself. I felt good about being able to help her in that process.

(Michael) My first professional massage was at a guy's house. It was so much work trying to make a relaxing environment. I was in *his* house and there were noises in the background that I knew were caused by his wife. We weren't able to separate the massage experience from the stresses in his life. I really wanted to work in a center at that point, a place where there was the right environment, the right pictures, the right flowers and so on. In my second massage I had found that place. But the first time was a big letdown for me. This client was basically interested in sex. Throughout the whole massage he kept trying to reach out and grab me. I said, "Wait a minute. It's got to be better than this."

Q. Is there any one type of individual you like to massage in terms of body type or tone?

A. (Marcia) I like to massage people who like to be massaged. Body type doesn't matter to me.

(Michael) I especially like to massage people who respond. There are some people who say they love it, but they don't really let go. The ones who really open up are good to be with.

Q. How can people make your job more enjoyable?

A. (Michael) Respond.

Q. What are some of your own techniques for helping your clients relax before and during the massage?

A. (Marcia) I have a brief talk that I give before the massage so they'll know what to expect. I'll tell them how I want them to lie and tell them to let me know if anything is uncomfortable. I'll explain briefly just what I'm going to do. I ask them if the room temperature is comfortable, if they feel comfortable and so on. During the massage, if there are some areas where they don't seem to be relaxing, I might direct them to use their breath in different ways to aid them in relaxing.
(Michael) Usually I'll reassure my clients and encourage them to let go, to take more responsibility as the massage progresses, rather than me doing it. I feel that my skill in helping a person let go has improved since I started working.

Q. How can someone best prepare for his or her massage?

A. (Marcia) A hot tub bath before the massage is great. Also, find the areas where you have the most tension and tell the person who is massaging you.
(Michael) You should be sure that you don't have anything planned for the rest of the day. You don't want to go back to a stressful environment. You don't want to be rushed to get there, either.

Q. How do you prepare the massage room?

A. (Michael) There's a whole science to that. One of the things we've always done is use white sheets on the table. Some people say, "No, no, it's too clinical. You will do better with tie-dyed sheets, something to remind your clients that they're doing something hippy or spiritual or counter-cultural." But we use white sheets because for us that's professional; it's clean. We want the room to look like a place a client can feel safe in. Usually we have music on. It's meditation music or classical, sometimes jazz.

Q. What have you learned about yourself through giving massage? About people?

A. (Michael) I've learned how people do let go, how they go from a fairly superficial, tense level to a fairly deep, open one. By watching people do that and encouraging them to do that, I feel like I've learned how to do that for myself. I feel much more able to be personal and pleasant with people now than I did twelve years ago.

(Marcia) I feel that I get a different perspective of people. When I see people on the street I get impressions of what they're like through their mannerisms and appearance. When I'm massaging someone I get a different viewpoint. I'm getting totally different information from a different level. Sometimes I realize that I've developed an impression of someone just from talking to them in the office. Then I'm massaging them and feeling that they are a different person in there. It's like the old saying: "You can't judge a book by its cover." I get the cover *and* the inside pages during a massage.

My feelings for that person change. I think much more that that person is okay. Sometimes people will come in and I'll be impressed by their personal limitations. Sometimes people annoy me or I feel a personality conflict with them, yet I can get an entirely new perspective of them during the massage, a more accepting, unjudging perspective. That external personality isn't there anymore and underneath is somebody else. I don't feel annoyed anymore and suddenly everything is okay.

(Michael) I suspect that that is what people cry about. Most of the time people they interact with react to their own vision of "Gee, isn't she uptight." Or, "Isn't she tense?" It's what you're describing . . . it's almost like the person is finally seeing who he or she really is. Somebody is with them at that level for a whole hour.

(Marcia) That acceptance is important. People with rotten personalities also want to be accepted underneath. How many times have you had somebody think you were a jerk (laughter) and you say to yourself, "I'm not really like that underneath. If only they knew." When you're getting a massage there's that opportunity for someone to see that you that's underneath. It's what people mean sometimes by compassion.

(Michael) The other phrase I hear a lot to describe that experience is that it is something like unconditional love.

4

A Full-Body Experience

The closest I had ever come to receiving a full body massage before writing this book was from my girlfriend, who had taken one class in the basics of massage, but she wasn't what you'd call an experienced masseuse. Nevertheless, I enjoyed the experience immensely, but then she could have given a massage with claws for fingers and I still would have savored the intimacy of being touched by someone I loved. That is the beauty of giving massage to a close friend. The shared emotions more than compensate for the lack of expertise you might have.

But when I took on the responsibility of writing a book on massage I knew I would need to "get in touch with my subject." To get a "feel" for the book I would have to have a full body massage from a professional practitioner. Very conveniently, The Massage Center in Palo Alto was nearby so I decided to have my first massage there, after checking out its reputation and finding everything above board. According to friends, there wasn't any hanky panky going on, i.e., no sex.

The event proved the high-water mark in the assembling of information for the book. Many of the notions I held about massage would prove totally false. I would soon find out more about myself, about my inhibitions for being touched and about massage as a uniquely personal encounter. Afterwards, my feelings about massage turned from skeptic to banner waver.

I entered The Massage Center expecting one of two settings—a room filled with naked women standing around waiting to be "chosen" or masseurs dressed in robes, long-bearded and looking for all the world like displaced gurus. The masseuses would be wearing earrings through their noses and flowers in their hair. Instead, I saw a conservatively furnished room, with several comfortable looking couches, a bookshelf filled with massage literature and a half-dozen portable massage tables,folded. It was all quite disarming. Sitting at a desk,The Massage Center Practitioner talked on the telephone.She was booking a massage with a prospective client. I noticed a closed door and guessed that the massage rooms were behind it.

I was somewhat hesitant because of my guilt feelings about being there and it probably showed. After all, why should I, who was raised by the Puritan work ethic—like so many Americans—spend my time and money on something so seemingly frivolous as massage? Why should I splurge on myself? It appeared to be a blatant act of self-indulgence; I still believe it is, although I can justify it now for the benefits of mental and physical well-being.

I told the woman at the desk that I was writing a book on massage and that I decided to see what it was all about, at least from the sensual side of massage. I figured that was a good reason.

The masseuse was pleasant enough and her accommodating attitude helped me relax. She wore a sweater and slacks, nothing suggestive. I talked about the book and told her what would be in it. She said that she would like to give the massage and explained that I would be her first client since returning from a three-month vacation in Japan. "My hands have gotten out of shape, so I hope I can make it through the day," she said smiling. Since I was there for a sensual massage and not physical therapy I didn't put much importance on her concerns. I was to learn later that giving massage requires considerable hand strength.

We arranged to meet at 6 p.m., right after I got off work. I was nervous. I told my fellow employees at Palo Alto Bicycles, where I work part-time, and everybody joked about it, tossing out sexual innuendos and asking me what type of sex I would ask for. I laughed and assured everyone that this was *not* a sex massage parlor. But I was learning that even my friends didn't understand the difference between sensual and sexual. To them massage *is* sex and there isn't any other way to look at it. I have decided to keep massage sessions strictly personal.

I went to The Massage Center well prepared, just in case my

friends were right and I had been misled. I wasn't about to take all my clothing off so I wore some nylon running shorts that would be comfortable, my symbol of modesty. My masseuse assured me that I could wear whatever I liked and made no effort to convince me I must have a nude massage, although she added that it is common practice. I was learning just what a prude I am.

I undressed in one of the massage center's four rooms after paying. The Massage Center is emphatic about payment in advance, and prefers that you make a deposit as an incentive to show up for your appointment on time. The room was about twelve feet by ten feet, with a massage table occupying most of this floor space. The walls were painted a bluish-white and had a couple of scenic posters. A shelf lined with massage lotions also had a clock. A shaded light on the ceiling lit the room brightly and the window shades were drawn. I had about five minutes to undress and familiarize myself with the ceiling as I lay on my back on the massage table. I felt like a patient waiting to be operated on while I contemplated my fate. The massage table seemed too narrow and prevented me from relaxing my arms. I could let them hang over the edge and look like a beached seal or I could keep them at my side and feel like a canned sardine. I decided to be a sardine.

Finally, the masseuse entered and quickly started working, first with my head, rubbing her hands through my hair and using a scented oil. I liked that part of the massage. As she stroked my neck I liked it even more. I was enjoying this sensuous massage, so far. My expectations of sexual exploitation took a back seat to the enjoyment of being touched, sensually.

I wanted to strike up a conversation with the masseuse, to tell her where it felt good or bad, but I held back. I was under the impression that a sensuous massage is conducted in silence (that is generally how it is done) and I didn't want to appear crude by babbling. But I found this communication blackout somewhat disturbing. Later, I was told that had I wanted to talk, it would have been all right. I should have clarified this aspect of the massage experience ahead of time. I was soon to learn that there were several other important matters I should have discussed before the massage began.

The masseuse continued pouring oil into her hands and rubbing it on my skin until it seemed like I might slip off the table. At least the room temperature was comfortable and I never felt chilled. She moved farther down my neck, taking long, soothing strokes from my shoulders up to my head, by way of the neck. I found this extremely pleasurable and wished she could have spent more time there. But this was a full body massage and I wanted to see what was in store for me elsewhere. The arms came next, but she did not touch my face. She lifted my arms and in a single stroke moved from the shoulder to the hand. She also worked on my hand, manipulating the palm and the fingers with gentle kneading. This was quite a pleasing technique, far more memorable than the arms.

About this time I had one thought in my mind: Relax! I kept telling myself to relax, to let my body turn into a blob of Jell-O, for two reasons—to further enjoy the massage and because I didn't want the masseuse to think that I was nervous. But my subconscious was waging a battle between ethics and basic needs and desires. Too many inhibitions and too much "body armor" had built up over the years—like barnacles on a rusty ship hull—to allow this complete stranger to touch my body in such a way. And yet it was enjoyable. Consider the impact of being touched sensually when for years you have been conditioned to see touch as sexual. Touching has fallen into clear, non-threatening patterns normally experienced by Americans: the doctor touches you for medical purposes; a friend pats you on the back or touches your shoulder; your mother or father touches you for family togetherness, and your lover touches you lovingly. But this person was touching me sensually, a complete stranger giving me sensations reserved only for those you are truly close to. And it was not sexual. This was confusing and I know it made me more uptight than I would be otherwise.

The masseuse worked next on my chest and stomach as I contemplated my position. The shorts probably prevented her from executing a full body stroke from chest to leg, but I was more concerned with appearing as non-sexual as possible and that meant remaining clothed. The closer she came to the area below my waist, the more thoughts crossed my mind, visions of massage parlors, perverse affairs repeated in the fantasies of millions of sex-starved Americans. (What the masses really are, though, is touch-starved.) Within each of us there must be enough imaginations to make a dozen pornographic movies. That's because so many of us have fallen victim to the *Playboy* mentality of sex, sex and more sex. As much as I might publicly claim my liberal attitudes and support of women's liberation, I was a male chauvinist pig. If our inner thoughts were to be revealed, how many times would they make hypocrites of us? I fought the emotions, but it was about as effective as Don Quixote doing battle with windmills. The beast within had been well trained by *Piayboy* brainwashing.

Before turning onto my stomach, the masseuse finished with strokes to the legs, using her patented long, smooth motions while applying generous pressure. I had always envisioned a sensual massage as light stroking, as lightly as possible without tickling. I noticed that the hair on my legs was being pulled and it felt uncomfortable even though the masseuse used liberal doses of oil. I had seen many movies where professional bicycle racers received leg massages from their masseurs and I realized then how important it was that they shaved their legs for a good massage.

I had decided on keeping my eyes shut as much as possible through the massage. It was a difficult decision, because I wanted to see her technique and yet I didn't want to make the masseuse feel self-conscious. I could simply close my eyes and pretend that I was enjoying the experience, but then muscles don't lie. She could tell I was tight. I decided to open my eyes only occasionally.

The masseuse finished my legs quickly and moved to my feet, where my remaining fears met their Waterloo. The big earthquake that will someday send half of San Francisco into the bay could have hit right then but I would have insisted, "On with the massage!" Here in the feet was bliss, ecstasy and intoxication. Most of our nerve endings find their way here, so the feet have an acute sensitivity. But normally our feet are on the receiving end of pain from blisters, calluses, sore arches and stubbed toes, and when someone does touch your feet for pleasure, they usually wind up tickling. But in the hands of a massage expert, watch out! I could have spent the remainder of the evening having my feet massaged. I didn't need a full body massage, I needed an hour of foot massage.

I told the masseuse in no uncertain terms how much I was enjoying her foot work. She smiled and said something about how most people have the same reaction.

She finished with my feet and asked me to turn onto my stomach. I wanted to tell her to forget the back and continue with the feet but decided in the interest of research that I should go through with the full body massage.

It might help you to know something about my feet. For ten years they have been those of a marathon runner. They've been driven relentlessly over thousands of miles of rock-hard pavement, jabbed unforgivingly into the shoe toes until blisters and calluses formed. They've been neglected and ignored. Now they were being treated to a sensation more exotic than anything I could have ever imagined. I urge, I plead for every runner to sprint down to the nearest massage center for a half-hour foot massage. It should be required treatment after a marathon. I can see the impact of runners getting a massage; the country will become hooked. Foot massage parlors will spring up everywhere, as quickly as car lots are going bankrupt. Long lines will form outside massage centers as runners wait for their turn.

But back to reality. And a harsh reality it would be after I turned over. The masseuse began with some long strokes over my back, which felt good. But then she discovered some knotted muscles near both shoulder blades and began drilling with her thumbs, which hurt so good. I know I got those knots from weekend bicycle rides of up to 130 miles. For every mile I traveled, hunching over the handlebars, the muscles got tighter until they were like tensed springs. The masseuse tried to uncoil them. I had suggested that she work on any tight muscles she found, especially in my legs, and that proved my undoing. I had come thinking sensual massage (of the Esalen ilk) but gave my masseuse instructions for physical therapy. Her thumb dug underneath my shoulder blade and I winced again. I knew she was putting everything she had into it; the weight of her body pressed against me. She twisted her thumbs back and forth and the pain worsened. I imagined this masseuse to be some shiatsu practitioner gone berserk. My face grimaced and I let out a soft moan. "Does that hurt?" the masseuse asked sympathetically. "Yes," I moaned. "Well, it's no wonder, there's a huge knot right where my thumb is. Just try to relax and breathe deeply." By now I wanted a stick between my teeth. The masseuse moved to work on my other shoulder, where she dug in with equal force. Massage is enjoyable, I kept reminding myself, but other less rational thoughts began seeping in. She reassured me that she was getting that nasty knot out and that I would feel much better the next day.

Just as suddenly as it had begun, it was over. The masseuse completed with a few more strokes on my head and then left the room so that I could dress. She said I could rest and not to hurry getting up.

I could have taken a shower, a convenience provided every customer, but I decided that since I was riding home, I wouldn't need one. With all that oil on my skin, though, I could have used it in the event I had to return to work.

I looked at the clock and noticed that a full hour had not passed. Taking into account the five minutes preparing for the massage and five minutes on this end, the actual massage lasted from fifty to fifty-five minutes. But I was amazed by how quickly the time seemed to pass.

I dressed and walked back into the reception room, where I greeted my masseuse. She asked me how I felt and I said "Fine." We said our good-byes and I rode home on my bicycle, feeling as though I had just finished a sixty-mile workout. My body felt like it was full of lactic acid and my shoulders were sore. I was feeling relaxed, though, as if I had drunk a couple glasses of wine.

Overall, I considered the experience a good one, but I had learned a few rules about massage and how to make it even more enjoyable next time. You must make clear to your masseur or masseuse just exactly what you want in the massage. That is the golden rule. Consider some other fine points: 1) If you want a sensual massage, be sure you ask for it. If you want physical therapy, let your masseur know something about how you think massage will help. Although massage is not a benefit of most insurance company policies, even as physical therapy, if you have a doctor's recommendation, it often will then be accepted by insurance companies. And most massage centers have at least one physical therapist. Even if you're there just to have your muscles rubbed, be sure you let your practitioner know about: 2) Setting. If the room seems cold or drafty, tell the practitioner. 3) Lighting. If a light bothers you, have it turned down or off. 4) Oils. Make your request ahead of the massage. There are many different kinds (see Chapter 6). 5) Talking. Some people like to talk to their practitioner. If you do, tell him or her. 6) Music. Most massage centers offer music for their patrons. It's usually piped in through stereo speakers and is always something melodic. 7) Clothing. This is your choice. Wear what you like, but don't expect to get a massage with all your clothes on. The point is, you don't have to do it in the nude.

I've pretty much decided on what kind of massage I like after just one visit. There's a foot reflexologist in town who gives a great massage. Sensual foot massage will be the coming rage. I plan on being the first one in line.

5

Body Maintenance

No doubt about it, a daily massage would make us healthier, happier people. But there is an insurmountable problem about this—logistics. Who is going to take an hour out of their day for a full body massage? Who will give you the massage? Only the extremely wealthy could afford to have a daily massage. So, we wind up getting a massage from a close friend or at a massage center when we can afford one. The vast majority of Americans have not even experienced a professional massage.

After reading this chapter you might decide to run right down to the nearest massage center and take advantage of a positive, even rewarding experience, both physically and emotionally. Just consider some of the reasons why massage benefits the body:

1) Increases local blood supply to joints
2) Hastens drainage from region of involved joints, thus decreasing periarticular swelling
3) Produces muscular relaxation
4) Increases lymphatic and venous return
5) Prevents fibrosis and adhesions in muscles and decreases the tendency toward muscular atrophy
6) Functions of the skin are improved
7) Blood is attracted to the surface from internal parts
8) Nerves are stimulated or soothed
9) Efferent matter is removed more quickly
10) Nutrition is increased
11) Massage is a pleasurable experience.

But before dealing with the benefits from massage it is important to understand the nuts and bolts of how the human body functions. Those who attempt to conduct a massage and who have no working knowledge of human anatomy are inviting trouble; in fact, they might even injure their partner, or at least cancel the potential good from a massage. Physical therapists and professional masseurs and masseuses are required to attend schools that teach massage and anatomy. A practitioner requires certification from one of these schools, to avoid just such a danger. While no harm will come from the simple and friendly stroking of a companion, say on the back of the neck or around the shoulders, massage takes on a greater complexity when the entire body is involved and different techniques are used. Once you have read this book you can be confident that you will have the necessary knowledge of massage and human anatomy to give a simple massage to a friend. The major systems—circulatory, nervous and lymphatic—will be described first and then the affect of massage on them.

CIRCULATORY SYSTEM

Man's survival is dependent on a very complex and amazing plumbing system that covers every square inch of his body; it is as intricate as the most complex computer system and must never spring a leak, at least for very long. The heart keeps the plumbing system going; it is the central organ, a muscle that by its contraction and relaxation pumps blood to all parts of the body through a network of arteries; the farther from the heart the arteries are, the smaller they become. The smaller artery networks are called arterioles, which in turn decrease in size to open into a close-meshed construction of microscopic vessels called capillaries. Blood carried in these arterials holds life-sustaining nutrients and oxygen, which are needed by the muscles and organs. Once blood completes its task and drops off its nutrients, it is collected into a series of larger vessels, called veins, by which it is again returned to the heart—carrying a wealth of toxins and carbon dioxide. This old blood will be revitalized in the lungs and sent back out to complete another circuit. It takes from eighteen to twenty-four seconds for a blood cell to make the complete circuit of both the systemic and pulmonary systems. The systemic and pulmonary systems make up the two main divisions of the circulatory system. The systemic serves the body as a whole, except for the lungs. The pulmonary carries blood to and from the lungs.

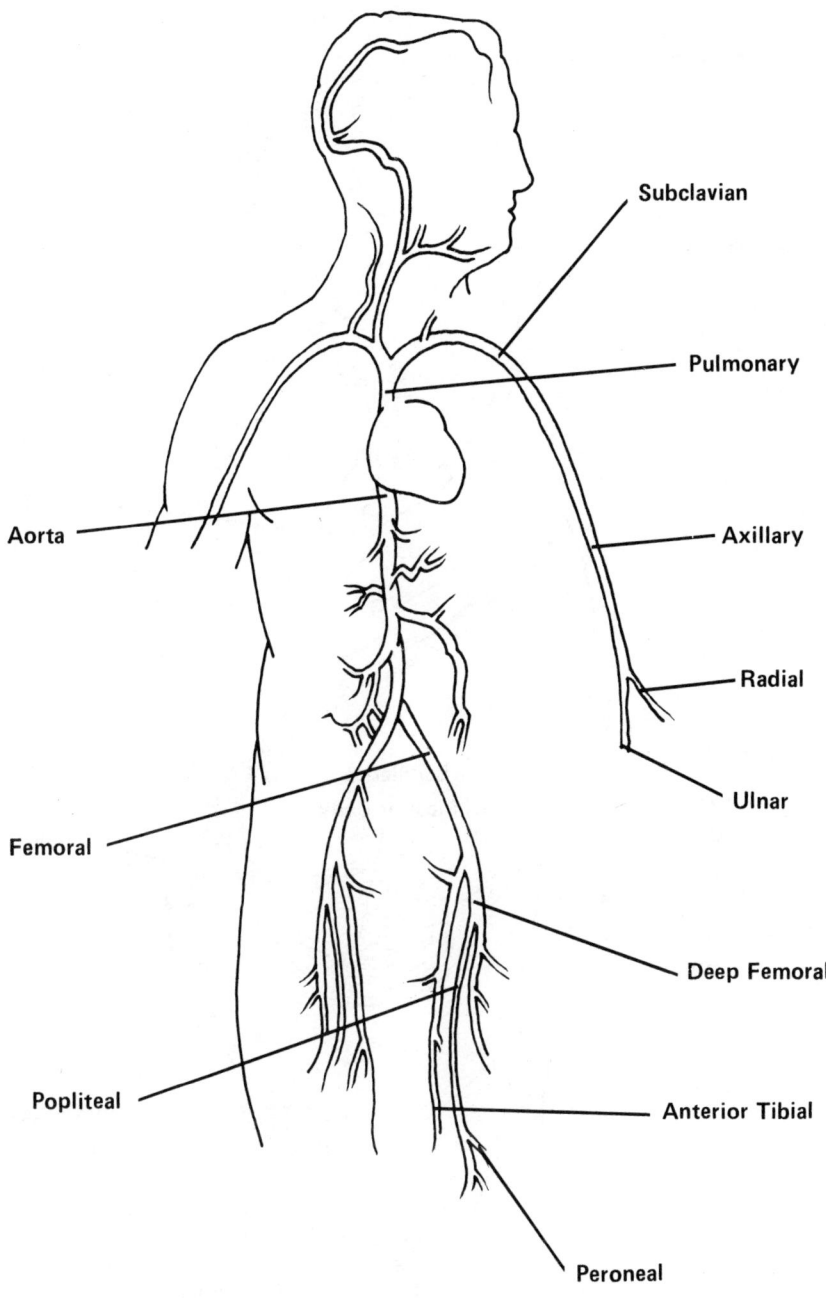

Subclavian

Pulmonary

Aorta

Axillary

Radial

Ulnar

Femoral

Deep Femoral

Popliteal

Anterior Tibial

Peroneal

Arterial Circulation

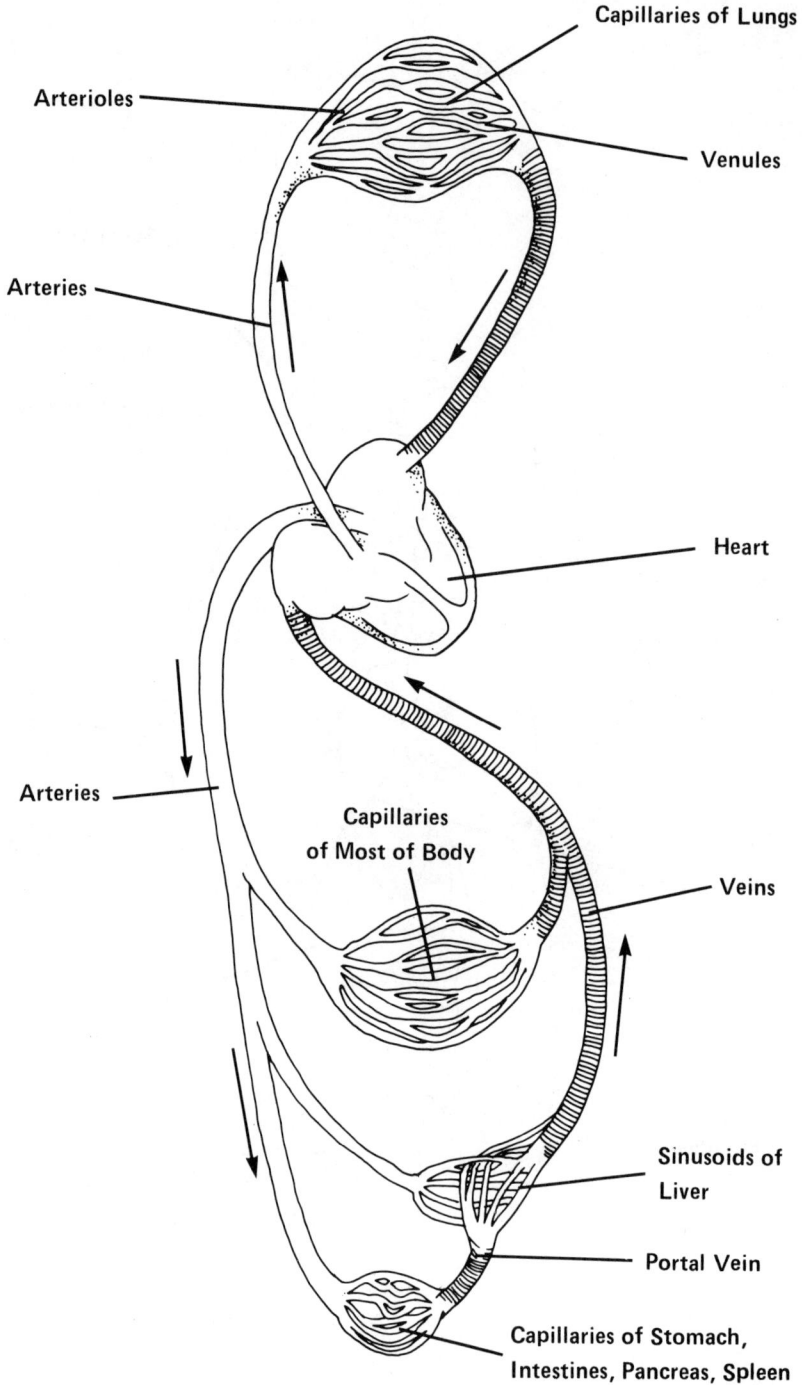

Capillaries of Lungs

Arterioles

Venules

Arteries

Heart

Arteries

Capillaries
of Most of Body

Veins

Sinusoids of
Liver

Portal Vein

Capillaries of Stomach,
Intestines, Pancreas, Spleen

Systemic Circulation

The heart is the only muscle in your body that can never rest. If it does take a breather, death is the result. The never-resting heart beats three billion times in the lifetime of someone who lives to age 70 and whose heart averages 80 beats a minute. With each heartbeat, two to three ounces of blood are pumped into the arteries. In terms of work, the heart lifts the equivalent of one ton to a height of 41 feet every 24 hours.

How does this amazing muscle work and what are its characteristics? It weighs about twelve ounces, less in women, and measures five inches in length, three and a half inches in breadth at the broadest point and is two and a half inches thick. It is divided in half, with a lower and upper chamber on each side. There are numerous valves throughout that keep the blood flowing in the right direction and prevent it from backing up or changing course.

The upper chambers of the heart are called the atrium and the lower chambers are called the ventricle. Blood circulation works like this: the right side of the heart receives all the venous blood and pumps it through the pulmonary arteries to both lungs, where it is oxygenated. The left side of the heart receives oxygenated blood from the lungs through the pulmonary veins. The blood is then pumped through the aorta and on to the entire body. Some of the blood returned by the veins enters the pulmonary circulation. After entering the right atrium and then the right ventricle it passes into the pulmonary artery. This is the only instance when an artery contains venous or dark blood (deficient in oxygen). The artery branches out in the lung into capillaries.

There is one important secondary circulation, involving the digestive system, called the portal circulatory system. The blood that moves through the spleen, pancreas, stomach, small intestine and the greater part of the large intestine is collected into a large vein, termed the portal vein, rather than heading directly back to the heart. It is carried instead to the liver. In the liver this vein divides, much the same way as an artery, and finds its way into capillary vessels, from which hepatic (liver) veins arise and they in turn carry the blood back to the heart.

MASSAGE AND SYSTEMIC CIRCULATION

Because the rapidity of the flow of blood depends on the difference between the arterial and venous pressure, any activity that can quicken the emptying of the vein must have a favorable

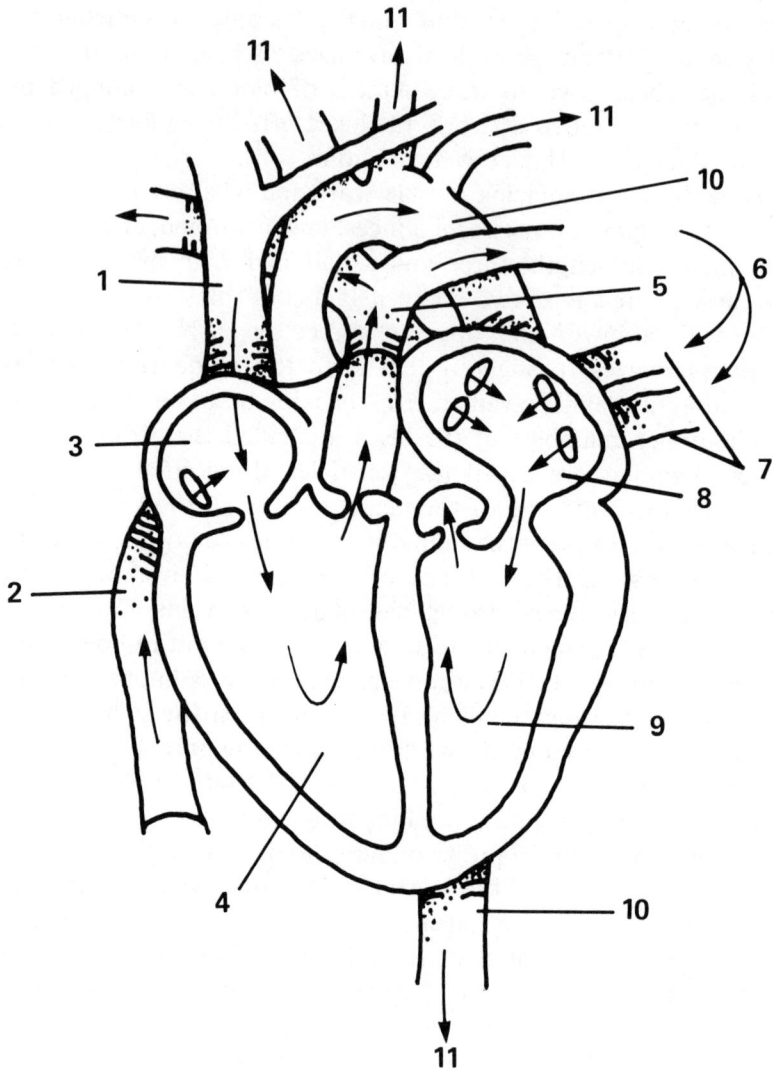

Heart showing course of the blood coming from the body and entering from (1) superior vena cava and from (2) inferior vena cava; to (3) right atrium; to(4) right ventricle; to (5) pulmonary artery; to (6) lungs (not shown); to (7) pulmonary veins; to (8) left atrium; to (9) left ventricle; to (10) aorta; leaving by (11) to the head, neck, and upper extremities (not shown).

influence on circulation. Massage does just that and, as we know, the better your circulation, the better will be your health. One test showing how massage increases circulation involved the injection of Chinese ink into the knee joints of a rabbit. One joint was massaged, the other left without treatment. On dissection, it was found that the joint massaged was empty of ink, while ink was still found in the other. The injected material was found in the lymph nodes of the massaged side, but none in the others.

If you've ever had a full body massage, you've probably experienced a feeling of drowsiness and complete relaxation. Or you've certainly petted a cat to the point that it begins purring and curls up in your lap for a rest. The stroking sensation of massage is most relaxing, but circulatory changes are also taking place. Centrifugal friction (rubbing down the body) diminishes the blood supply to the brain, and hence lessens cerebral activity. You can even obtain relaxation of the deep-lying organs by using light friction over them. This increases the activity of the overlying vessels and causes blood to go around instead of through the organ.

Massage can work to reduce mental fatigue through its affect on the circulatory system and the eliminative organs. The toxic substances produced by mental activity are more rapidly oxidized and removed from the body by massage, while the hastened blood current more thoroughly repairs and cleanses the wearied nerve tissues. What better therapy can the tired, overwrought business executive ask for, after a grueling day at the office, to promote relaxation than a full body massage?

In response to the demand for more blood to parts of the body being worked, the heart rate increases slightly, but it does not raise the arterial tension, as does exercise. Not only is circulation increased in answer to the greater demand for the removal of the poisons resulting from oxidation, as in exercise, but through the mechanical assistance afforded by massage, in moving the blood forward in the venous and lymph channels, and in setting up reflex activities whereby the small vessels are dilated and their activities quickened. This so-called "pump" effect of massage is something that must be learned to be effective because you need to know which way to stroke in order to get blood moving in the desired direction. For example, immediately following an injury it is important to reduce swelling and decrease circulation to the region. In this case you will want to stroke lightly away from the area. But after a day it is then important to increase circulation to the region and you will want to stroke toward the area, to hasten the removal of tissue waste and bring in new blood to speed the healing.

The increase in blood flow is usually accompanied by inflammation of the skin, so don't be alarmed if your partner's skin turns red in certain sensitive areas. Your partner might also notice an increase in warmth, sensibility, general vital activity and respiration. This is attributed in part to massage bringing into circulation waste products requiring elimination through the lungs and in increasing oxidation production, which necessarily accompanies the increased heat production resulting from the effect of massage upon the muscles. That's why your partner might experience a sensation of warmth. Massage can cause a rise in body temperature amounting to several tenths of a degree Fahrenheit. Using friction can actually increase heat elimination in the muscles by nearly 95 percent, according to author John Kellogg in *The Art of Massage*. Red blood cell production, according to Kellogg, goes up anywhere from 3 to 7 percent and, amazingly, anywhere from 40 to 80 percent in white cells.

The type of massage movement used and the location worked will affect the way your circulatory system reacts. Light percussion of the skin causes contraction of the blood vessels of that portion worked on. Strong percussion quickly produces dilation of the blood vessels, which can lead to paralysis in extreme cases. Light percussion, if sufficiently prolonged, also produces dilation. Basically, friction affects the superficial veins, while percussion works more directly on the deeper vessels. In terms of location, if you massage the abdomen, your partner's pulse will be slowed because of a raising of the general blood pressure; this is accomplished both by stimulation of the abdominal muscles, thus increasing the intra-abdominal pressure, and also by the stimulation of the vasoconstrictors of the abdominal vessels. Massage the legs and the portal circulation is acted on more directly, while massage of both extremities favorably influences the pulmonary circulation, in case of congestion of the lungs. With experience you will find how your massage of certain areas influences the mood and feelings of your partner. Then you can spend more time on the areas that bring the best results.

LYMPHATIC SYSTEM

In terms of plumbing, the lymphatic system can be compared to

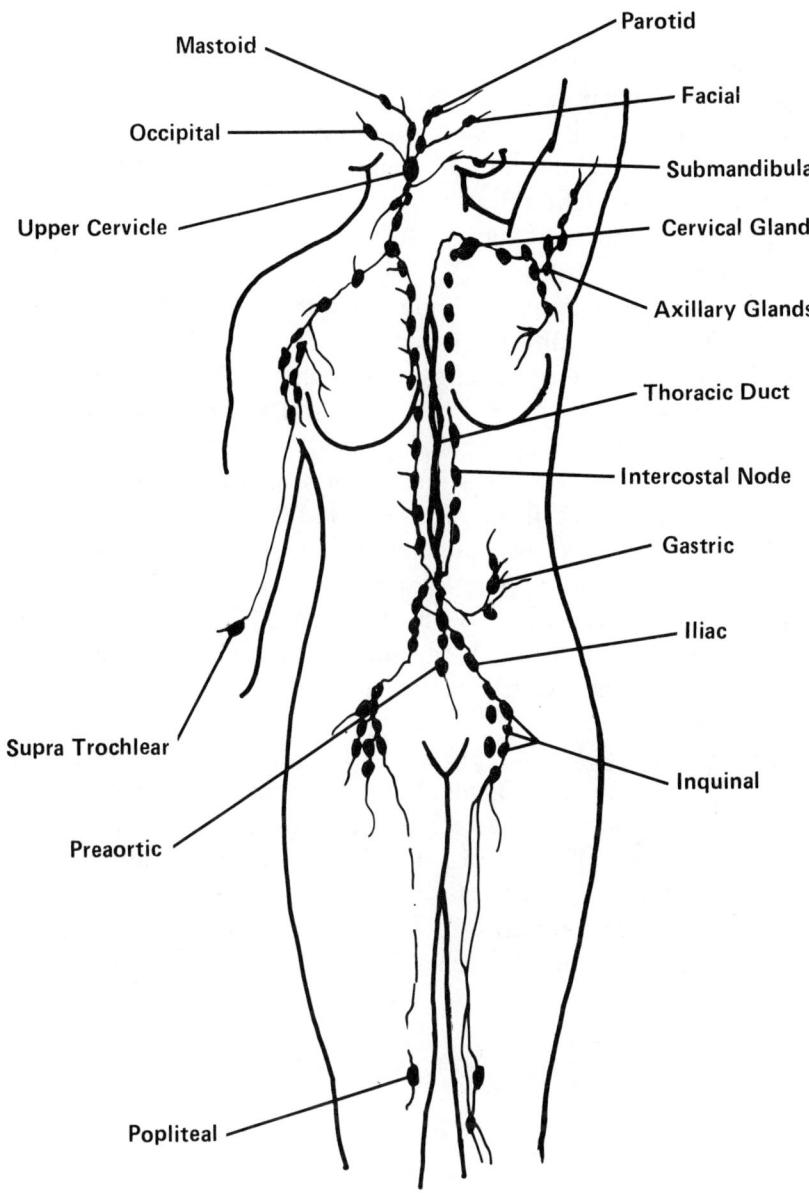

Mastoid

Parotid

Occipital

Facial

Upper Cervicle

Submandibular

Cervical Glands

Axillary Glands

Thoracic Duct

Intercostal Node

Gastric

Iliac

Supra Trochlear

Inquinal

Preaortic

Popliteal

Lymphatic System

the sewer lines in our major cities. It consists of a network of vessels, capillaries, nodes and ducts that serve to absorb and transport harmful bacteria and waste products. Lymph is formed in tissue spaces all over the body and is gathered into microscopic vessels that carry it centrally. All lymph eventually enters either the thoracic duct or the right lymph duct. The right lymphatic duct drains the right side of the head, neck and trunk and right upper extremity; the thoracic duct drains the remaining portion of the body.

Along the course of the lymph vessels there are lymph nodes, which function as filtering structures. They can be compared to the water treatment facilities, into which all sewer pipelines drain. They filter out bacteria and particulate substances that were left behind by the blood. A good location to actually feel one of these lymph nodes is just under your jaw bone about two or three inches back from your chin. It feels like a knot beneath your skin. Nodes can become enlarged (as big as an almond) during times of infection. The lymph node under the jaw becomes inflamed whenever there is an infection anywhere in the head or when you're down with the flu. It is a sign that your lymph system is working overtime capturing toxin.

Lymph is a kind of blood plasm, only without the red blood corpuscles. It is clear in appearance and has a lower protein content than red blood. The nodes are aggragated in regions, the principal ones being in the neck, the armpit and the groin.

Lymphatic capillaries arise in all parts of the body that are supplied by blood. They begin in the spaces of the connective tissue and form networks all over the body. The larger trunks follow the deep blood vessels; their walls are similar to those of the veins, but thinner.

MASSAGE AND LYMPH CIRCULATION

Lymph circulation, like the blood, is readily influenced by massage. In fact, you can even have a professional lymph massage. The lymph system is so sensitive to massage because lymph channels are most abundant just beneath the skin and in the fascia, which cover and lie between the muscles. These lymph vessels are thus mechanically acted upon in massage, especially by friction and kneading.

Experiments have shown that the flow of lymph from a limb in a state of inflammation is very easily induced and is seven or eight times greater than from a sound limb. Additionally, a swollen limb is known to diminish during the flow of lymph. And direct massage of a lymph node increases the outflow of the fluid. It stands to reason that the greater the flow of lymph, the better prepared your body is to resist infection.

NERVOUS SYSTEM

The nervous system is both man's blessing and his tormentor. Toothache pain is one of the most agonizing pains because it is rooted in the sensitive nerve endings of the affected tooth. But a far worse pain, one that no amount of morphine will relieve, is caused from skin burns. Millions of delicate nerve endings in the skin that are damaged by fire heal slowly and painfully. Yet the nerve endings that cause us such misery are also responsible for the exquisite sensations of loving. Whether for pain or pleasure, all of our senses are tied directly into the nervous system. The nervous system keeps us in touch with our world and its unending multitude of sensations.

The nervous system consists of the brain and spinal cord (which together form the central nervous system) and the peripheral nerves. The living tissue of the nervous system begins with a nerve cell, or neuron; they branch out into thread-like structures called dendrites. The peripheral nervous system carries nervous impulses to and from the central nervous system. Efferent fibers (nerves that carry messages from the brain) carry impulses to the muscles and other parts of the body that respond to stimulation. The peripheral nervous system consists of the cranial nerves, the spinal nerves and the sympathetic nerves. The spinal nerves arise in the spinal cord, thirty-one pairs radiating to either side of the body. They include nerves that control our senses, facial expressions, tongue, and so on.

The autonomic nervous system is concerned with control of involuntary bodily functions; it regulates the function of glands, especially the salivary, gastric and sweat glands, the adrenals, smooth muscle tissue, the heart, lungs, digestive organs and blood vessels. It may act on these tissues to reduce or slow activity or to initiate their function. In special cases, certain individuals have gained control over their autonomic nervous systems. According to Michael Nash, author of *Runner's World Weight Control Book,* skilled yogis, practitioners of Hatha Yoga, have learned to regulate

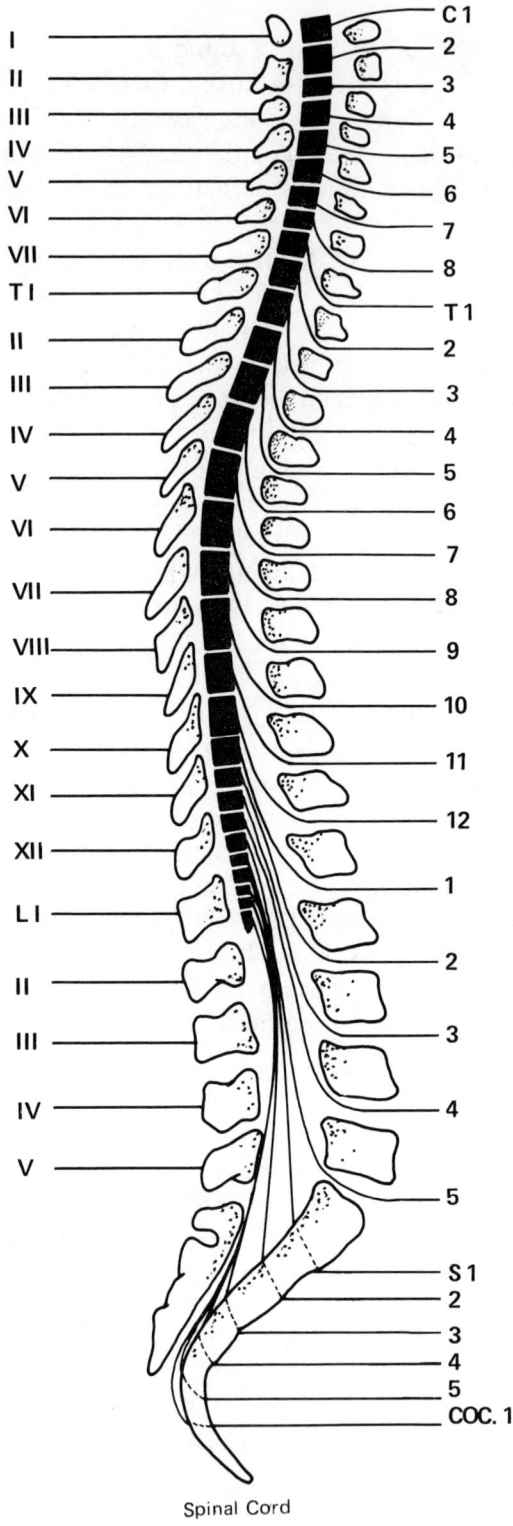

I

II

III

IV

V

VI

VII

T I

II

III

IV

V

VI

VII

VIII

IX

X

XI

XII

L I

II

III

IV

V

C 1
2
3
4
5
6
7
8
T 1
2
3
4
5
6
7
8
9
10
11
12
1
2
3
4
5
S 1
2
3
4
5
COC. 1

Spinal Cord

heart rate, respiration and bleeding. Yogis can lower their body metabolism to 50 percent of normal. During sleep the body's metabolism drops only 10 percent of normal. To do this requires intense concentration and years of practice.

In order to maintain the proper balance or function in the organs it controls, the autonomic system is comprised of two networks of nerves, the sympathetic and parasympathetic, which have opposing actions. For example, stimulating the sympathetic fibers usually produces vasoconstriction in the part supplied, general rise in blood pressure, erection of body hair and goose bumps. But stimulation of the parasympathetic system produces vasodilation of the part supplied, a general fall in blood pressure, contraction of pupils, slowing of the heartbeat, and so on.

We commonly associate all of our actions, such as hitting a baseball with a bat, with stimuli originating from the brain, which is generally true, but there are important exceptions. There are instances when the time it takes for a dangerous sensation to reach the brain and for the brain to send out the appropriate response signal, however fast it may seem, isn't quick enough to avoid injury. For example, when your hand touches a hot stove you instantaneously withdraw the hand. This is not a response made by the brain—the signal never reaches it. Instead, a motor nerve cell takes over. Motor nerve cells are scattered throughout the body and are what cause reflex actions, such as the withdrawal of your hand from the hot stove.

MASSAGE AND THE NERVOUS SYSTEM

The sense of touch is perhaps one of man's most influential and emotional feelings. It can evoke pain or pleasure. Massage is on the pleasurable side when it stimulates nerve endings on the skin in a pleasing manner. It brings a sense of well being that is impossible to simulate through drugs or other artificial means. The type of massage motion you use can also bring a variety of responses from the nerves. Light stroking or friction will relieve muscle tension by soothing reflex nerves, which is similar to the effect of petting a cat. But if you stimulate the nerves through pounding or heavy friction and kneading, the nervous system is going to react differently and register increased blood flow, perhaps even pain if the pounding is with sufficient force.

There are nerve endings and nerves in the body that call for particular caution when massaging, most notably on the elbow, also known as the "funny bone." It gets that name because the ulnar nerve runs through the elbow very close to the skin surface. Jarring or giving a sharp blow to the elbow sends a sensation, not unlike an electric shock, through the arm, although there may be very little true pain. Other sensitive areas include the groin, the ears, the face and the feet. Stroking too lightly in these regions will tickle.

MUSCLES

Muscles are readily identifiable and conjure up all kinds of thoughts at their mention. They are the pride of bodybuilders, the bane of high-paid female models, the source of our strength and a painful reminder, when they are overworked, of our humanness.

We are about 75 percent muscle and without them our skeletons would be no more than a bag of bones, unlike the insects, which have their skeletons outside of their bodies. Muscles are also distinguished by their ability to give mobility, through their contractibility. There are two muscle types, voluntary and involuntary. Voluntary muscles are normally controlled by the will and are attached to the skeleton. Involuntary muscles are beyond our control; they propel the contents of the stomach and intestine and the blood in the circulatory system. Some muscles work both voluntarily and involuntarily; for example, breathing can be controlled at will but also goes on mechanically during sleep. The heart muscle is odd in that it is constructed like a voluntary muscle (striated) but is involuntary in action.

The involuntary muscles have a smooth, nonstriated structure. Their cells are usually arranged in sheets or layers, but may occur as isolated units in connective tissue. The striated, skeletal muscles are voluntary muscles and are grouped in bundles called fasciculi, each of which is surrounded by a sheath of connective tissue called perimysium.

A typical muscle consists of a central fleshy portion or belly and its attachments. One end, called the head, is attached to a fixed structure termed the origin; the other end is attached to a moveable part called the insertion. Muscles may be attached directly to the bone or by means of tough cords of connective tissue, called tendons.

Muscles fall into two categories of movement, abduction/adduction and extension/flexion; muscles that draw away from the body centerline are called abductors and muscles that draw toward the body are called adductor. Extension is the separation of two muscles or body parts, while flexion is the movement of one body part toward another.

With 650 muscles in the human body (the number varies slightly according to which authority you refer to) almost all of them are aligned in pairs; for every muscle that works in one direction, there is a muscle that opposes it and moves in the opposite direction. An obvious example: the so-called biceps and triceps of the arm.

MASSAGE AND MUSCLES

Most massages are aimed at the muscles because they are the easiest part of the body to get to and respond so dramatically. That's because muscles receive most of their blood supply when they are moved. When muscles are inactive, blood seeks the easiest course by going around rather than through them. But massage emulates exercise by moving muscles and thereby increasing blood supply, just as exercise may be considered a form of massage, through the pressing and rubbing of muscles against one another.

When properly administered, the manipulation of massage acts upon muscles in such a way as to produce a suction or "pump" effect, pressing onward the contents of the veins and lymph channels, and thus creating a vacuum to be filled by a fresh supply of blood. The effect can be so dramatic that, according to author John Kellogg in *The Art of Massage*, "The increased blood supply of the muscle induced by massage naturally improves its nutrition. Experience shows that, when systematically and regularly employed, massage produces an actual increase in the size of the musculature structures. The muscle is also found to become firmer and more elastic under its influence."

Kellogg goes on to write that massage does have its limitations, though. "Massage feeds a muscle without exhausting it, in which respect it differs from exercise; nevertheless, it is not a complete substitute for exercise, because exercise brings into active play the whole motor mechanism—nerve center, nerve and muscle—while massaging chiefly affects the muscle."

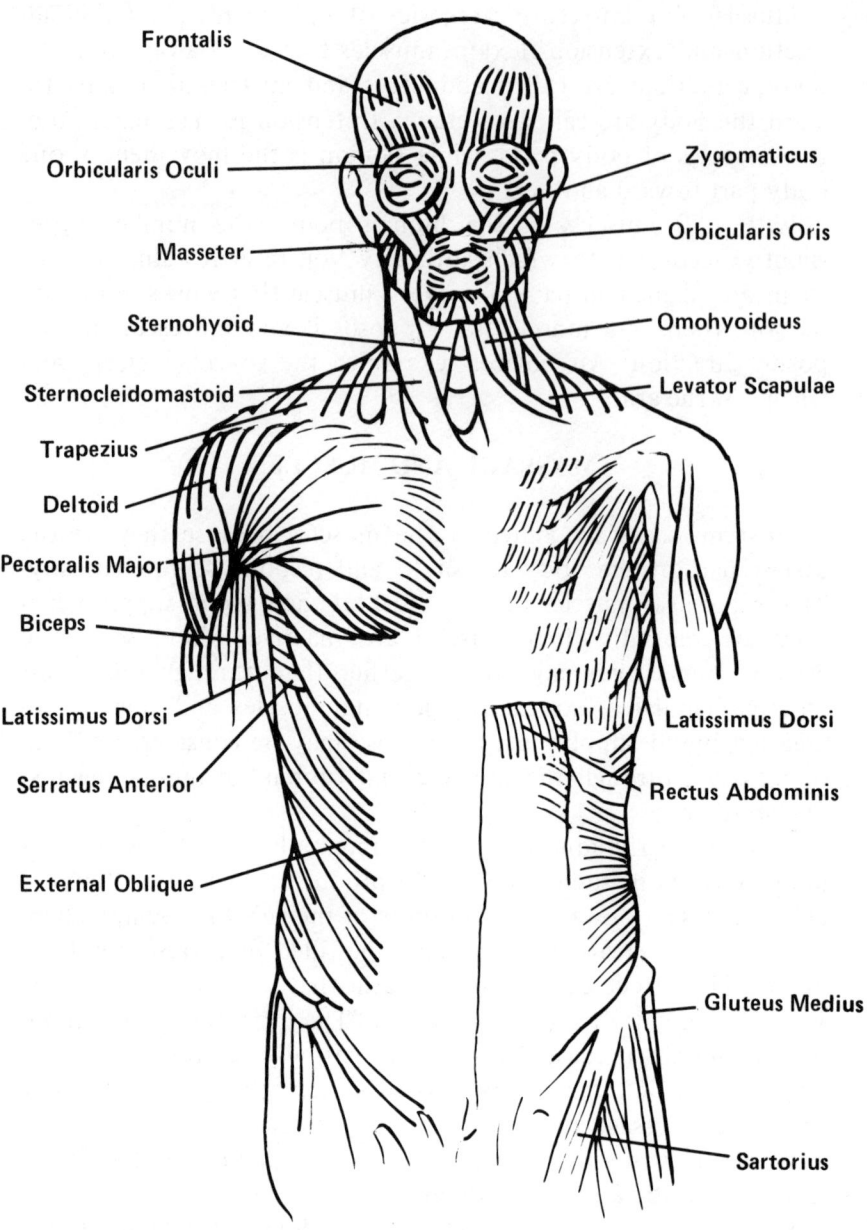

Torso Muscles, Anterior

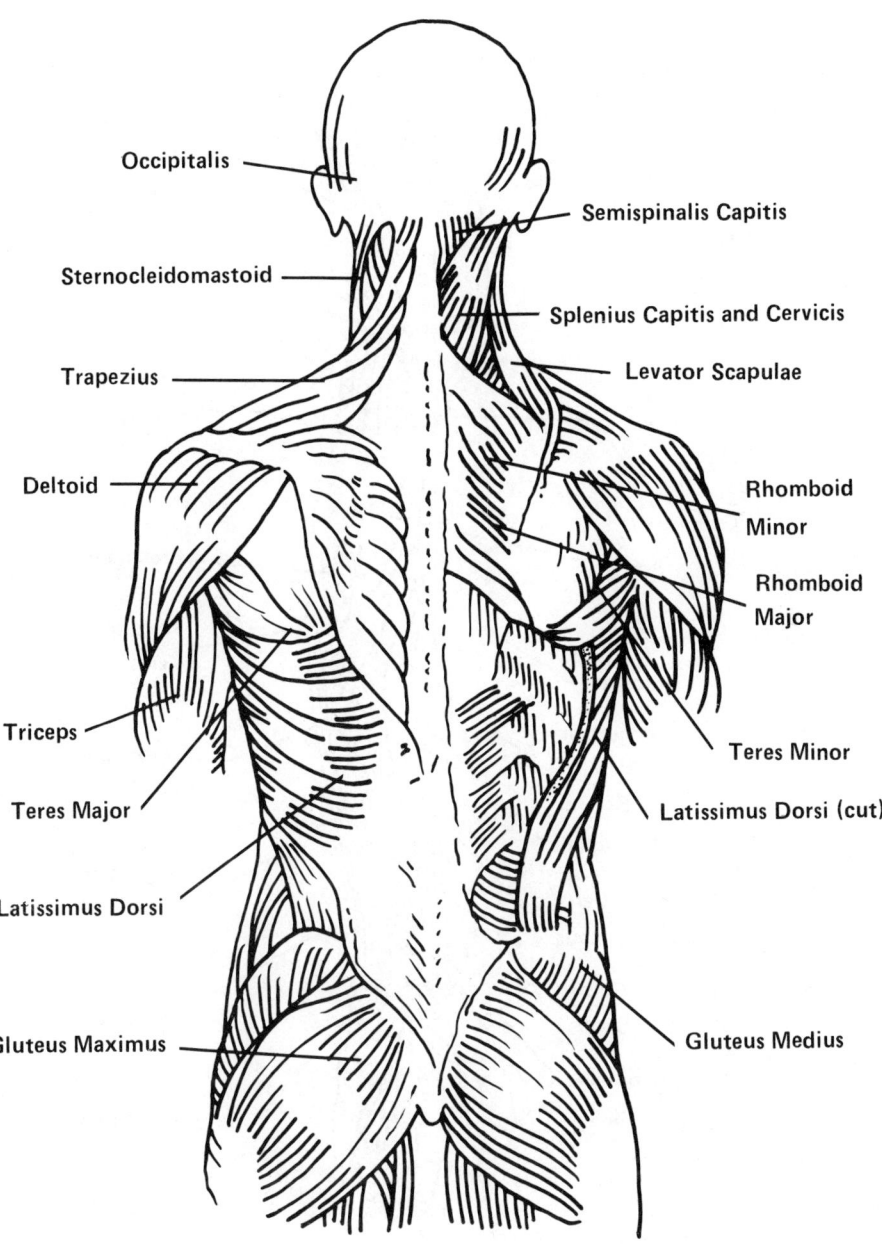

Occipitalis

Semispinalis Capitis

Sternocleidomastoid

Splenius Capitis and Cervicis

Trapezius

Levator Scapulae

Deltoid

Rhomboid Minor

Rhomboid Major

Triceps

Teres Minor

Teres Major

Latissimus Dorsi (cut)

Latissimus Dorsi

Gluteus Maximus

Gluteus Medius

Torso Muscles, Posterior

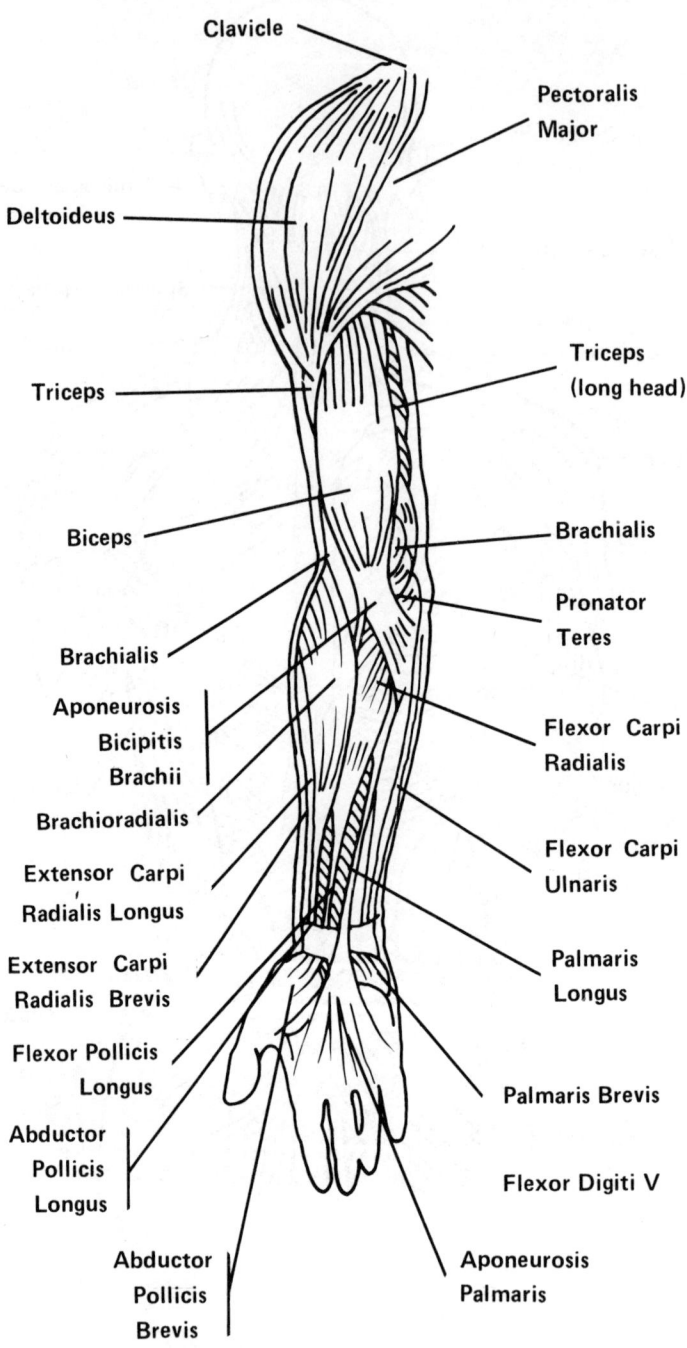

Clavicle

Pectoralis
Major

Deltoideus

Triceps
(long head)

Triceps

Biceps

Brachialis

Brachialis

Pronator
Teres

Aponeurosis
Bicipitis
Brachii

Flexor Carpi
Radialis

Brachioradialis

Extensor Carpi
Radialis Longus

Flexor Carpi
Ulnaris

Extensor Carpi
Radialis Brevis

Palmaris
Longus

Flexor Pollicis
Longus

Palmaris Brevis

Abductor
Pollicis
Longus

Flexor Digiti V

Abductor
Pollicis
Brevis

Aponeurosis
Palmaris

Surface Muscles of Right Upper Limb, Anterior

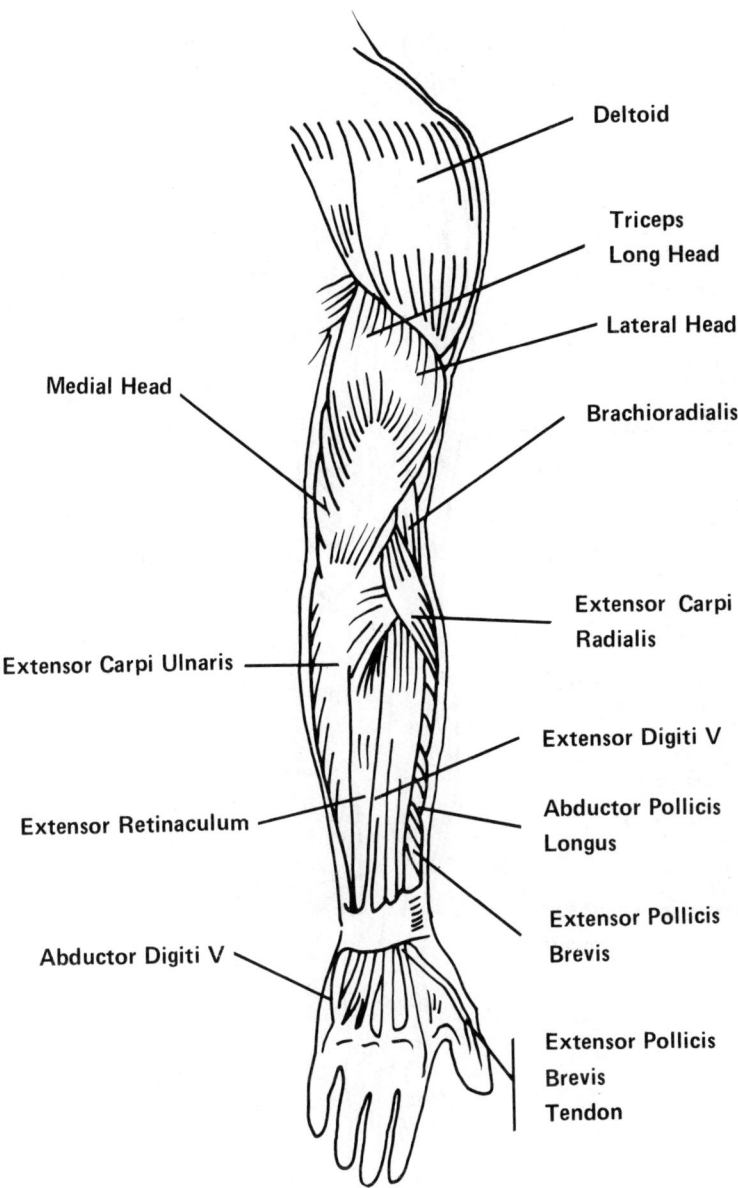

Deltoid

Triceps
Long Head

Lateral Head

Brachioradialis

Medial Head

Extensor Carpi
Radialis

Extensor Carpi Ulnaris

Extensor Digiti V

Abductor Pollicis
Longus

Extensor Retinaculum

Extensor Pollicis
Brevis

Abductor Digiti V

Extensor Pollicis
Brevis
Tendon

Surface Muscles of Right Upper Limb, Posterior

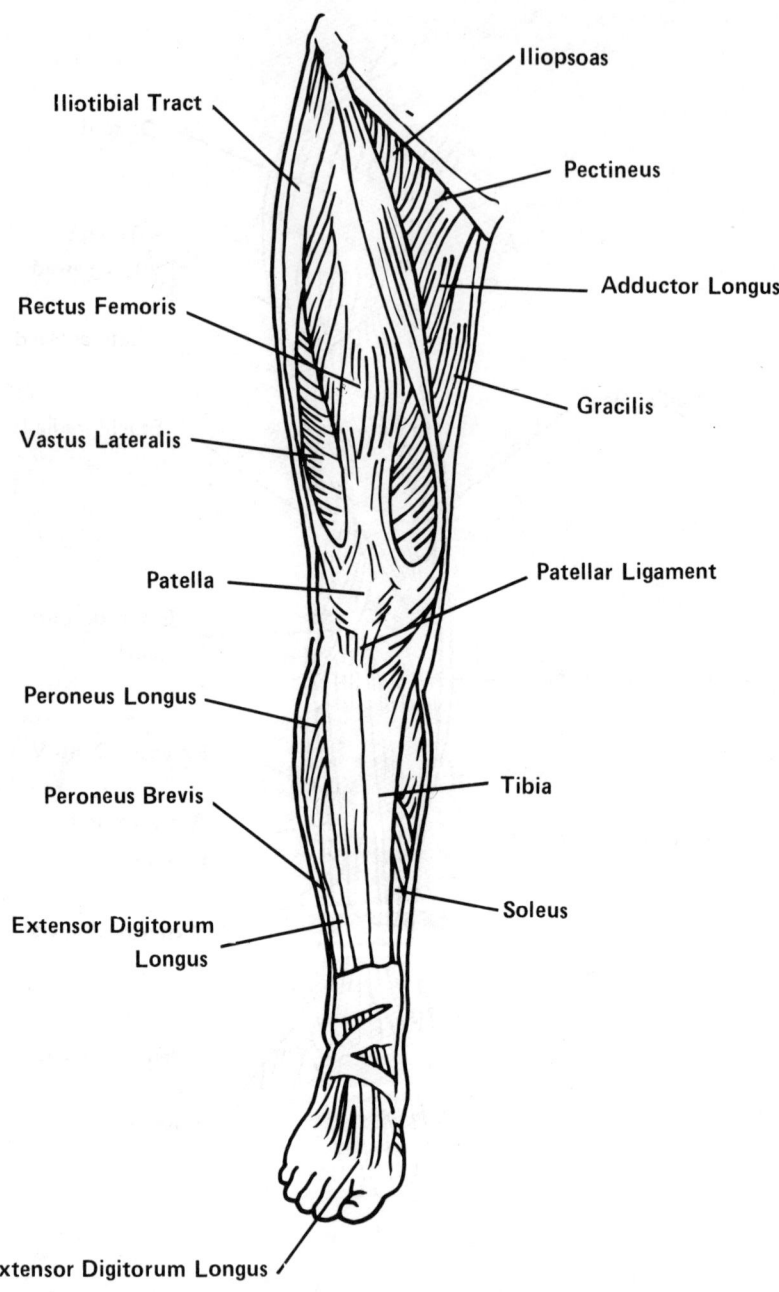

Iliotibial Tract

Iliopsoas

Pectineus

Rectus Femoris

Adductor Longus

Vastus Lateralis

Gracilis

Patella

Patellar Ligament

Peroneus Longus

Peroneus Brevis

Tibia

Extensor Digitorum
Longus

Soleus

Extensor Digitorum Longus

Surface Leg Muscles, Anterior

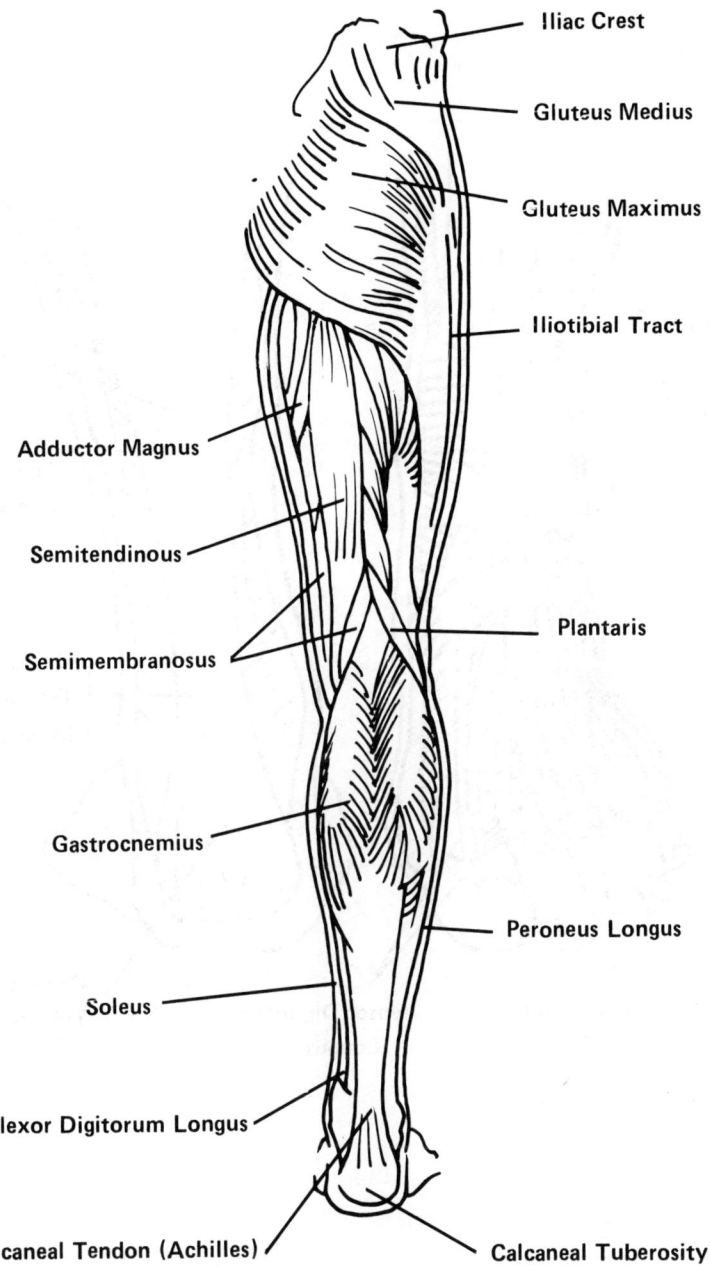

Iliac Crest

Gluteus Medius

Gluteus Maximus

Iliotibial Tract

Adductor Magnus

Semitendinous

Plantaris

Semimembranosus

Gastrocnemius

Peroneus Longus

Soleus

Flexor Digitorum Longus

Calcaneal Tendon (Achilles)

Calcaneal Tuberosity

Surface Leg Muscles, Posterior

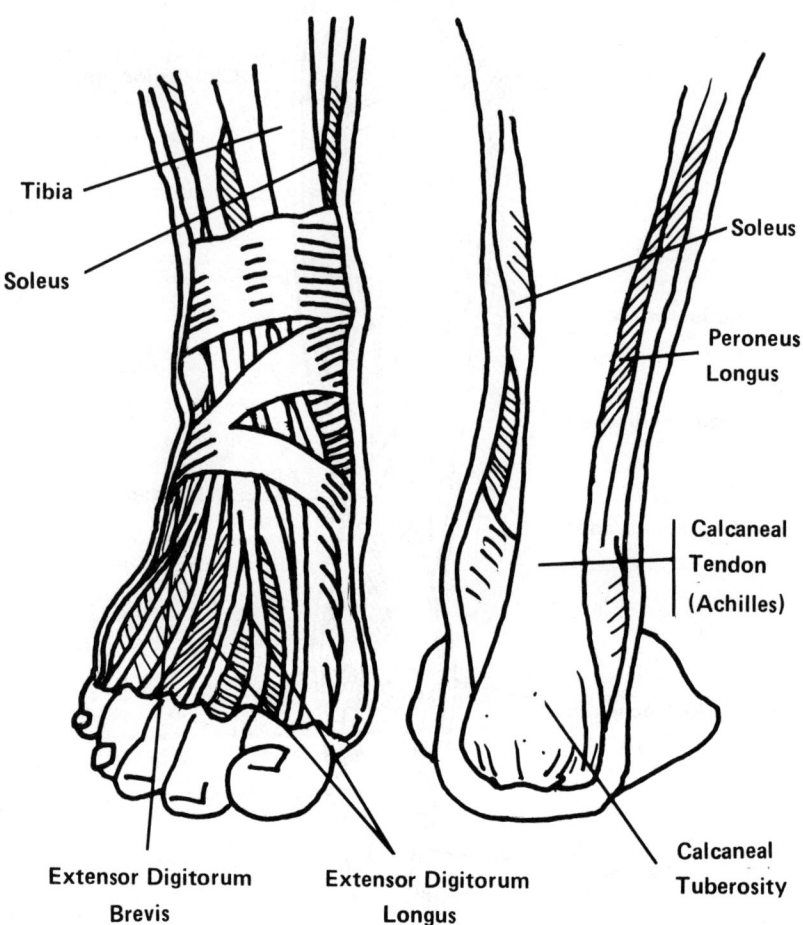

Tibia

Soleus

Soleus

Peroneus
Longus

Calcaneal
Tendon
(Achilles)

Extensor Digitorum
Brevis

Extensor Digitorum
Longus

Calcaneal
Tuberosity

Superficial Muscles of the Right Lower Limb

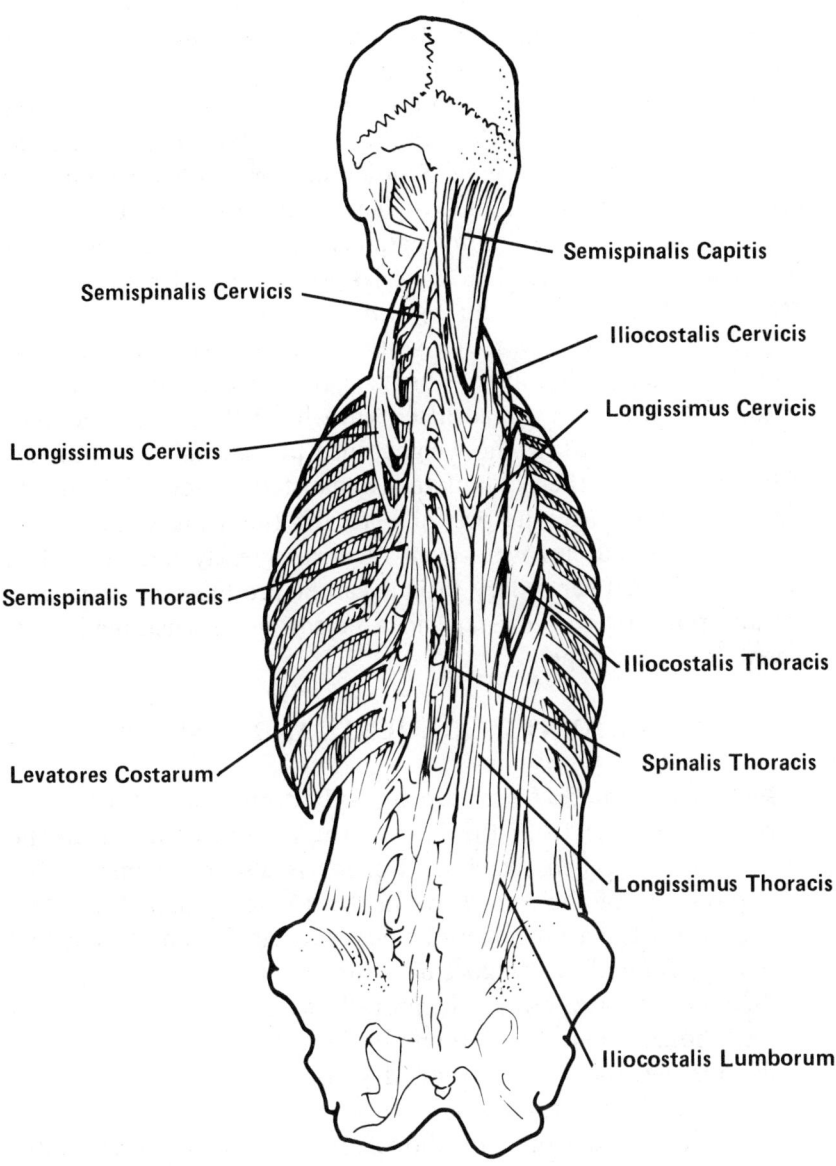

Semispinalis Capitis

Semispinalis Cervicis

Iliocostalis Cervicis

Longissimus Cervicis

Longissimus Cervicis

Semispinalis Thoracis

Iliocostalis Thoracis

Spinalis Thoracis

Levatores Costarum

Longissimus Thoracis

Iliocostalis Lumborum

Deep Muscles of the Back

Importantly, massage does not produce lactic acid as a by-product of exercising muscles. In fact, massage will help rid your muscles of lactic acid more quickly, after exercising for instance. Lactic acid plays a large part in muscle fatigue, which is why, after two hours of play, you are unable to hit the tennis ball as hard as you did in the opening serve. Studies support the statement that massage can help rid muscles of lactic acid. In one study, frogs were completely exhausted by paradization of the muscles. After fifteen minutes of rest their muscles were still not restored, but after a brief massage of the legs they revived at once and were even able to do twice as much work as before. Another test, this time conducted with human subjects, gave the same result, according to Kellogg: ". . . a man lifted with his little finger, one kilogram 840 times, lifting the weight once per second. The muscles of his finger were then completely exhausted. After a five-minute massage of the finger he was able to lift the same weight 1100 times and his muscles were even then not greatly fatigued." But be reminded that secondary fatigue can be produced by too vigorous an application of massage in a person not accustomed to it, or who is out of shape.

BONES, JOINTS, LIGAMENTS AND TENDONS

Bones are what give the human body form, all 206 of them. They range in size from the largest, the femur in the leg, to the tiny ear bones, called ossicles. "Bones" is also the name of the head physician of the *Enterprise* in the TV series *Star Trek*. And you can learn the arrangement of bones by singing an old spiritual tune, "Dry Bones," which goes like this:
Them bones, them bones, them dry bones,
Them bones, them bones, them dry bones,
Them bones, them bones, them dry bones,
I hear the word of the Lord.
Ezekiel connected them dry bones, Ezekiel connected them dry bones,
I hear the word of the Lord.
Toe bone connected to the foot bone, foot bone connected to the ankle bone,
Ankle bone connected to the leg bone, leg bone connected to the knee bone,

Knee bone connected to the thigh bone, thigh bone connected
to the hip bone,
Hip bone connected to the back bone, back bone connected to
the neck bone,
Neck bone connected to the head bone,
I hear the word of the Lord.
Them bones, them bones, going to walk around,
Them bones, them bones,
Going to walk around, them bones, them bones,
Going to walk around, I hear the word of the Lord.

A bone has a lot more life and fluid in it than you might think.
It is lined with numerous minute veins and nerves. Its interior is
filled with the very important marrow, a red or yellow substance
that produces many of our red blood cells. A bone, despite its
strength, is composed of half water.

As we grow older our bones become more brittle. In youth
they are as pliable as rubber, which explains why so few children
break bones when they fall. But in old age, bones become brittle
and are broken easily. Keep this thought in mind when massaging
the elderly.

Bones are held together by thick, fibrous tissue called ligaments.
Tendons are similar to ligaments and they connect bones and muscles. The Achilles tendon is the strongest and largest of the tendons, attached to the heel and extending up the calf. A ligament
is pliant and flexible, designed to allow the most perfect freedom
of movement, but strong, tough and inextensile, so it won't yield
readily under the most severely applied force. But the tendon is
devoid of elasticity. It is very sparingly supplied with blood vessels, as well as nerves.

Where there are ligaments and tendons you'll usually find
joints. Where the joint is movable, ligaments and tendons play the
vital role of supporting the limb's mobility. There are several
varieties of joints, including gliding, ball-and-socket, hinge and
pivot joints. The ball-and-socket joint allows for the most movement, as in the hip and shoulder. The elbow is a hinge joint,
capable of only back-and-forth movement. A pivot joint occurs
where one bone rotates around a projection of another bone, as
the radius on the humerus. Bones that glide on each other are
called the gliding joints—the wrist for example. Joints are further
aided in their mobility by a smooth layer of hard tissue called

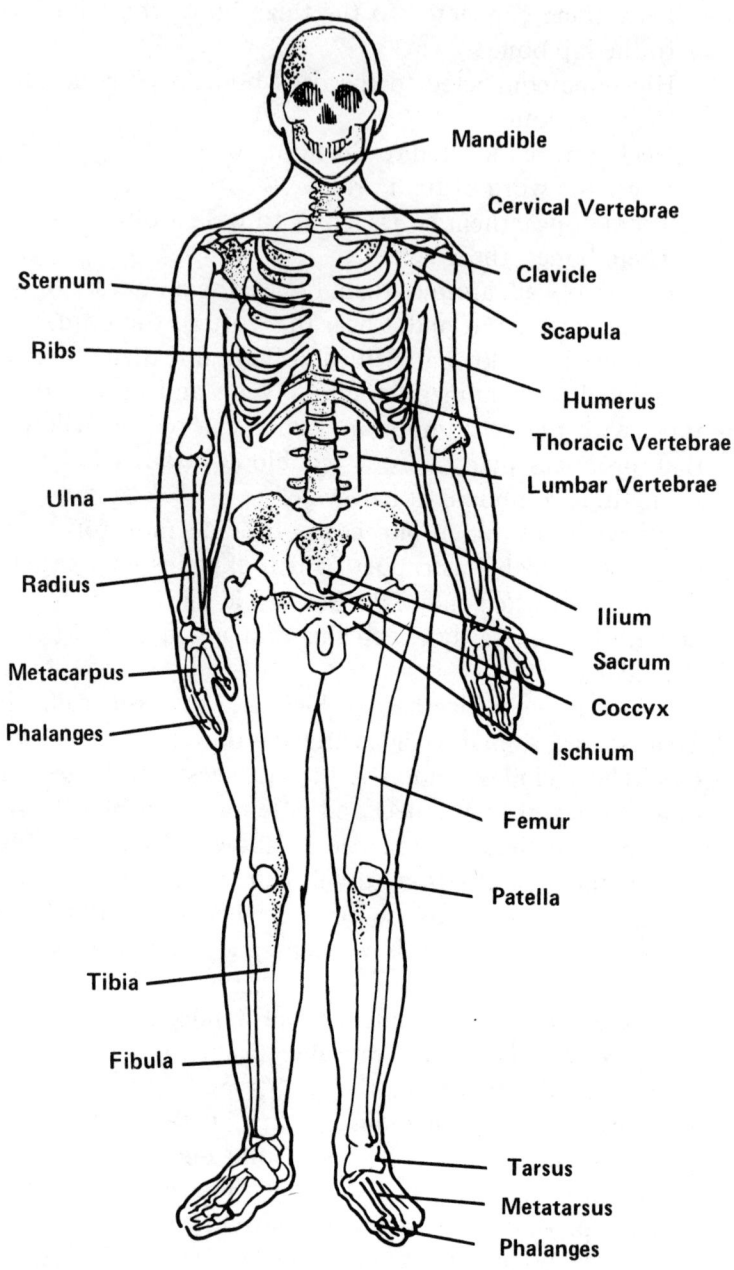

Human Skeleton, Anterior

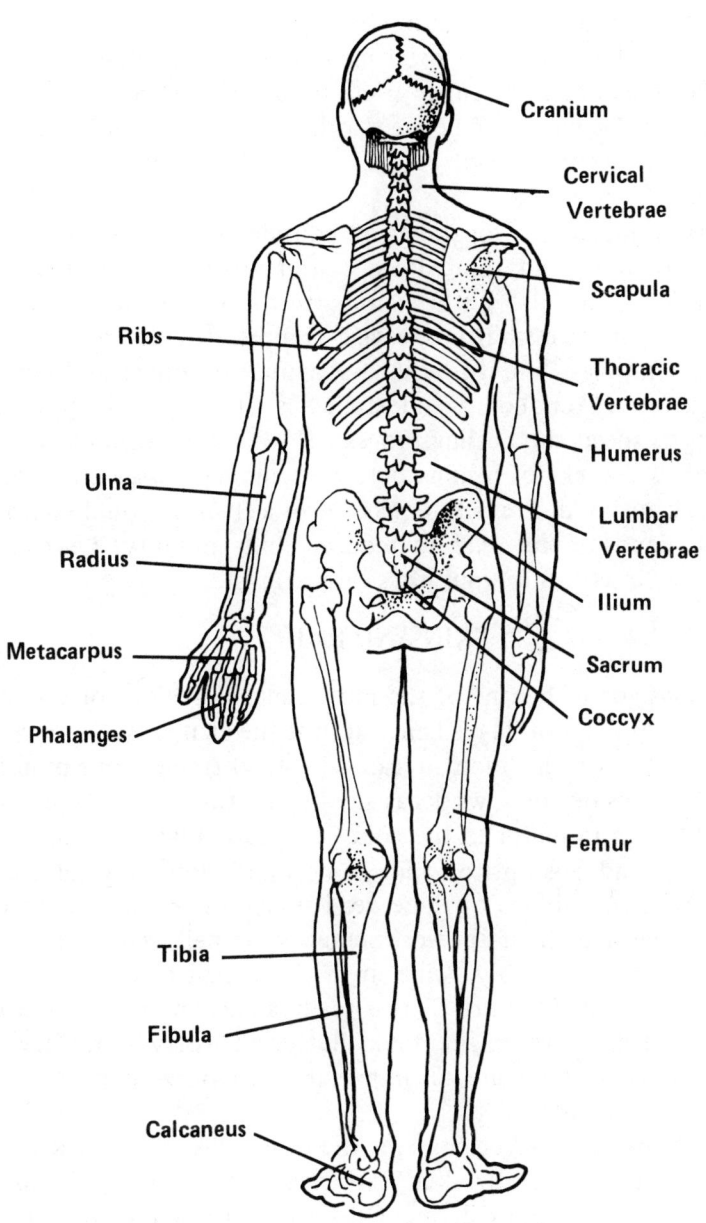

Human Skeleton, Posterior

cartilage, which is in turn covered by a clear liquid called synovial fluid. Synovial fluid is sometimes concentrated in a padlike sac or cavity found in connecting tissue, usually in the vicinity of joints. It is lined with synovial membrane and contains a fluid, synovia, which acts to reduce friction between tendon and bone, tendon and ligament, or between other structures where friction is likely to occur. Several bersae are located around the patella (kneecap).

Because joints are locations of considerable stress, they are subject to injury—anything from a strain to a torn ligament or tendon. They are also hotbeds for arthritis and rheumatism. Because of their accessibility, massage is most effective for circulation and muscles, but it is still of some use on bones and joints. Massage of broken bones and strains is often used in physical therapy to speed the healing process. However, you should give a fracture two weeks of healing before beginning massage, to allow the break to bond. Premature massage of a fracture could increase calcium deposits and lead to reduced limb mobility. Leave the massage of fractures to your physical therapist.

SKIN AND HAIR

Skin has got to be one of the most amazing regions of the human body because of its resiliance against the elements. No thicker than the skin of an onion, it can withstand tremendous punishment. It keeps out rain, works as an air conditioner in hot weather and acts as an insulator in the cold. It is both a living, vital organ (excretory and absorptive) and an accumulation of dead cells. Daily, we shed millions of these dead skin cells. We lose many of them during a bath or shower. Scrape your nail against the wet skin and you'll probably come up with a small amount of gray matter that looks like dirt. This is really an accumulation of dead cells, not dirt as you might think. But don't worry about having dead skin cells; they are an important part of your protection against the elements.

The skin's outer layer contains the dead cells and is called the epidermis, but the "true skin" is beneath this thin layer and is known as the corium or derma. On the surface of the corium are the sensitive papillae (little bumps) and within are the organs with special functions, such as sweat glands, hair follicles and sebaceous glands. The epidermis varies in thickness from the very thin eyelid, to the often callused palms of the hands and heels of the feet. It prevents the evaporation of water from your body. The hair and

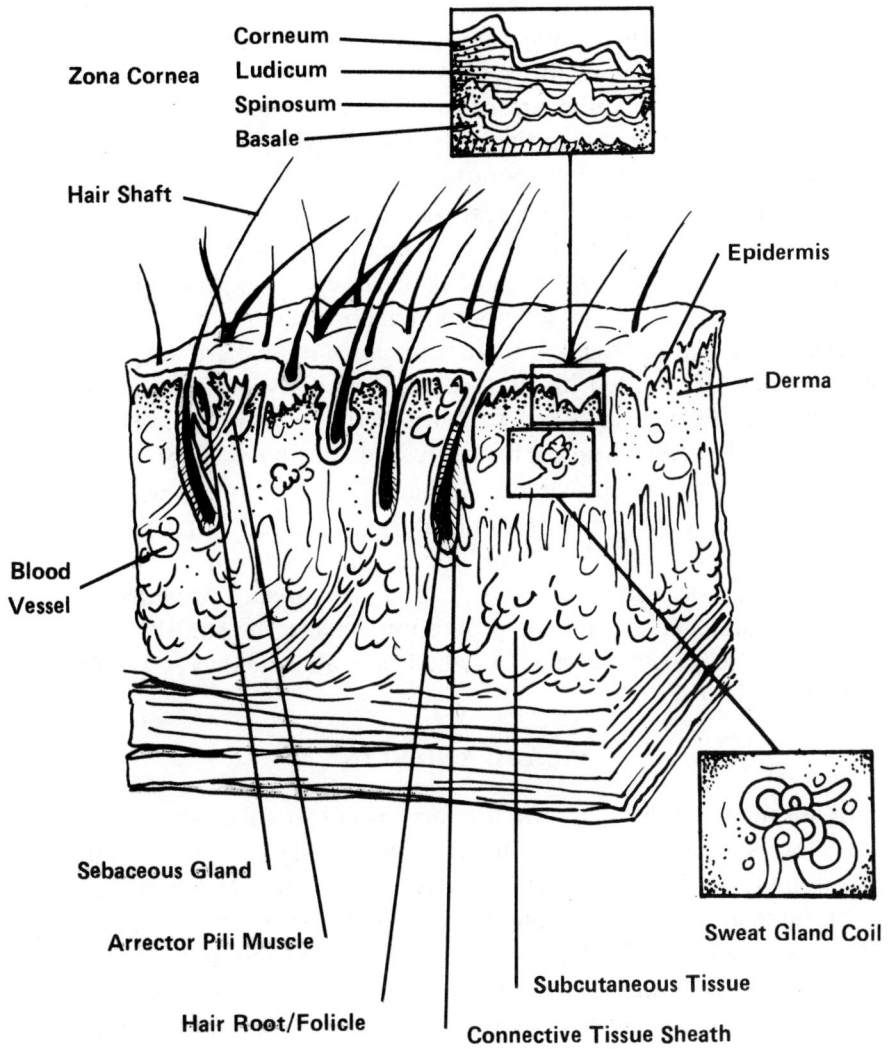

Corneum

Zona Cornea   Ludicum

Spinosum

Basale

Hair Shaft

Epidermis

Derma

Blood
Vessel

Sebaceous Gland

Arrector Pili Muscle

Sweat Gland Coil

Subcutaneous Tissue

Hair Root/Folicle

Connective Tissue Sheath

Layers of the Skin

nails are part of the epidermis and consist exclusively of dead cells, without nerve endings.

The corium contains all the important metabolic elements, such as lymphatics, nerves and nerve endings, blood vessels, sebaceous and sweat glands. Within each papilla is a capillary loop that furnishes the epidermis with a blood supply. Hairs are lodged here in what are called follicles and they cover almost every part of the body. Also important in this region are the sweat glands, situated in small pits on the undersurface of the corium. There are at least two million sweat glands in the body, but the whole of these glands would only represent an evaporating surface of about eight square inches. Of course, it is the sweat glands that help regulate body temperature on a warm day, by opening up and allowing perspiration to cover the skin and thus cool the body on exposure to air.

It is crucial for sweat glands to remain free of clogging substances. A running friend learned that lesson the hard way one summer day. He coated his body with a thick layer of suntan lotion before the run to avoid sunburn. After two miles he began noticing that he was heating up badly and that he was not sweating as heavily as he should be. He barely made it home without falling victim to heat prostration; later, he figured out that the suntan lotion was responsible for blocking his sweat pores.

My friend was not aware that nature has already provided us with a natural oil, sebum, for protection against the sun. It is secreted by the sebaceous glands, which are almost always associated with a hair follicle.

MASSAGE AND SKIN

Skin and its nerves are the primary receptors of massage. Not only does skin act as a transmitting agent through the nerves, but according to Kellogg in *The Art of Massage*, it is acted upon directly by massage. Oil production increases and hair growth is stimulated, especially on the arms and legs. Hartvig Nissen, in his book, *Practical Massage and Corrective Exercises* goes one step further in describing the influence of massage on skin and hair growth: ". . . there is no doubt, to my mind, that the *circular kneading* of the scalp will produce new growth of hair . . . The simple reason is that the massage will bring nourishment to the roots of the hair and thereby awaken nature to new life." Nissen even gives evidence in describing the success of massage on returning hair growth to a bald 65-year-old woman. Massage may stimulate hair growth but it cannot alter a genetic inevitability. If your genes

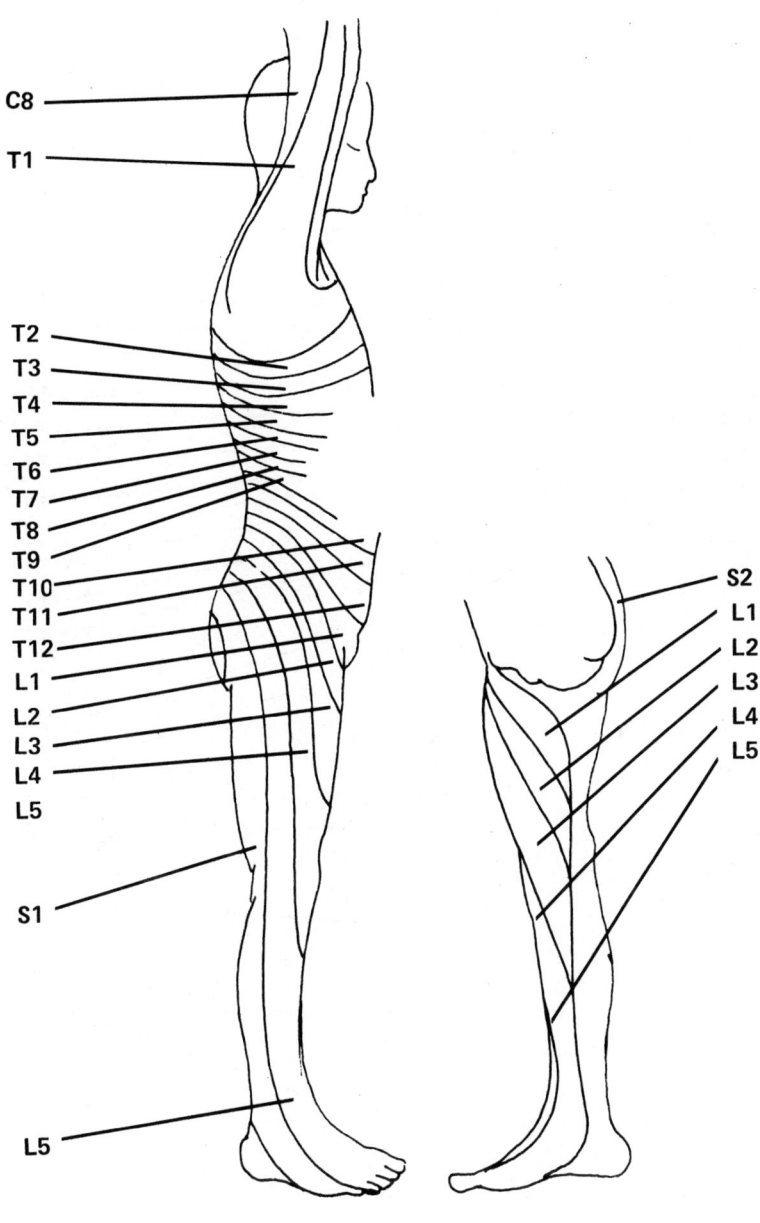

Dermatomes of the Upper and Lower Limbs

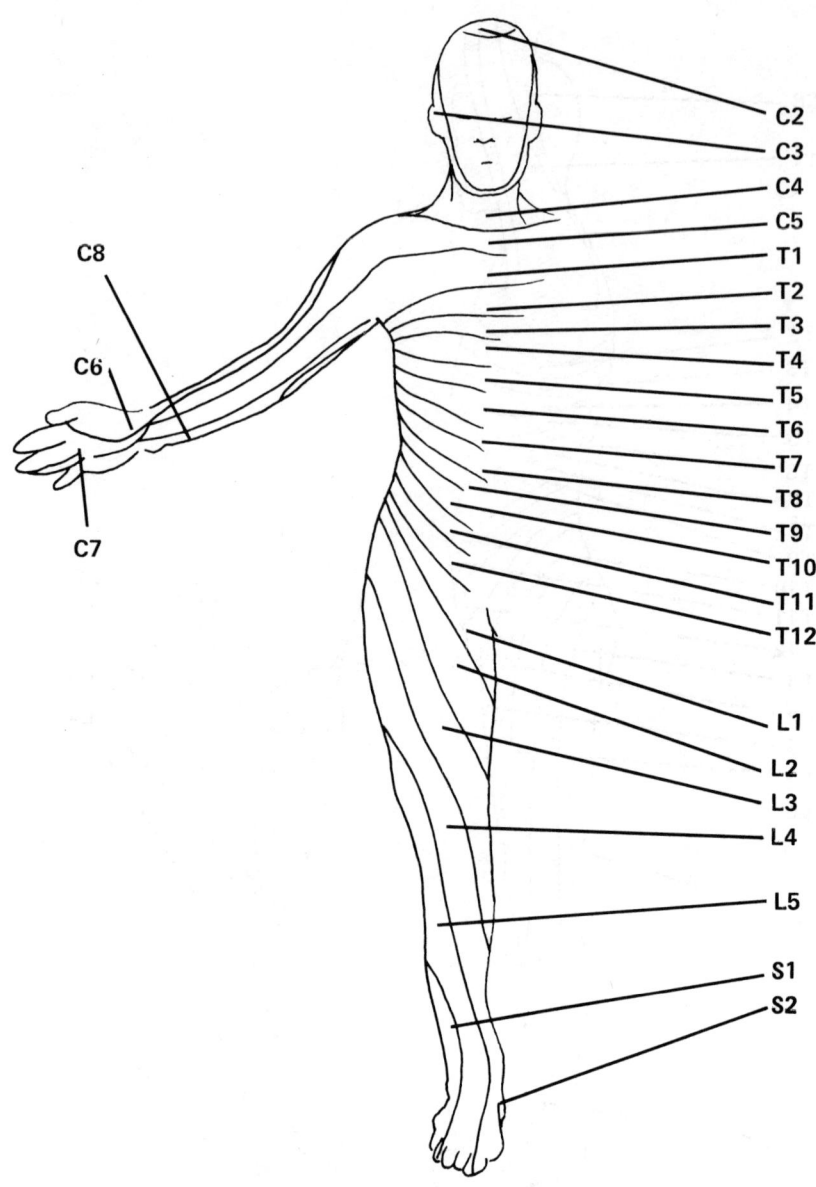

Dermatomes of the Upper and Lower Limbs

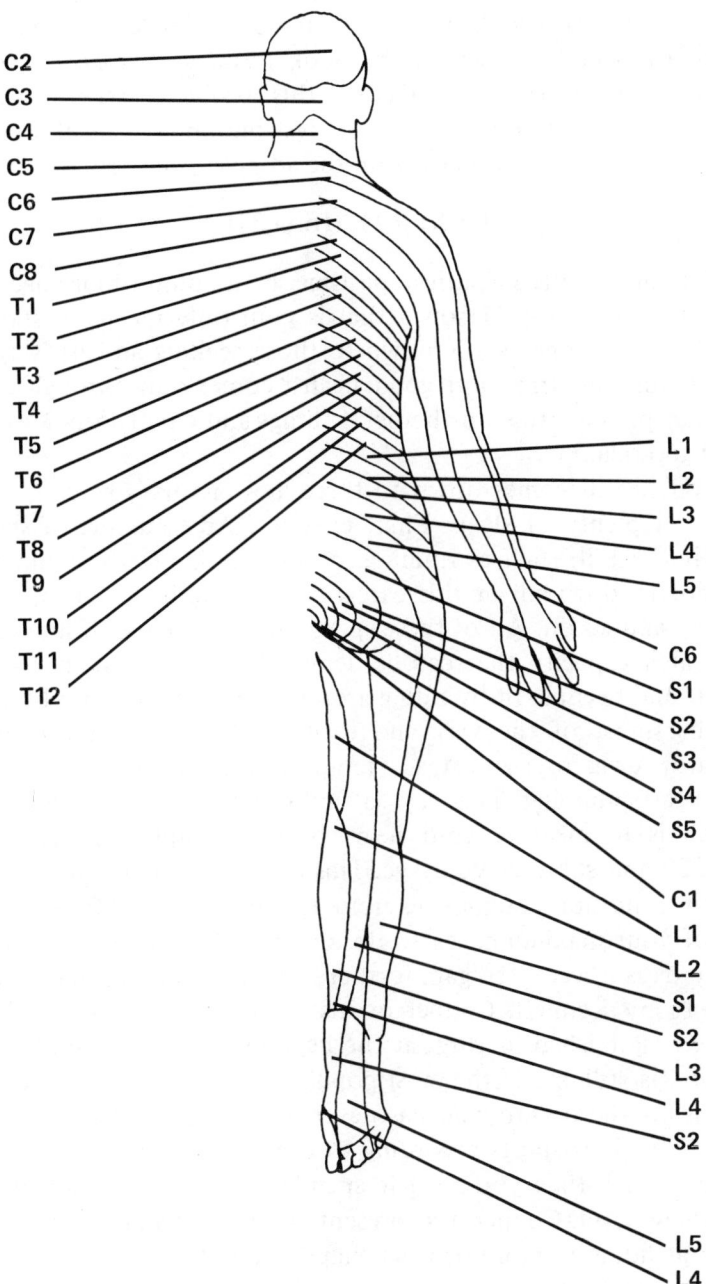

C2
C3
C4
C5
C6
C7
C8
T1
T2
T3
T4
T5
T6
T7
T8
T9
T10
T11
T12

L1
L2
L3
L4
L5

C6
S1
S2
S3
S4
S5

C1
L1
L2
S1
S2
L3
L4
S2

L5
L4

Dermatomes of the Upper and Lower Limbs

are on track for seeing baldness by age thirty; there's not much you can do about it, beyond getting a hair transplant.

In case you're wondering about what massage does to fat, you dieters had better look elsewhere for your miracle cure. According to Dr. Frank Krusen in the book *Physical Medicine*, "When Rosen [a physician] investigated this problem experimentally he found that vigorous massage of the abdominal wall of animals produced no destructive effect on the adipose [fat] tissue."

GENERAL HEALTH

While massage is a healthful pastime, no amount of massage will make you a healthy person if that is your only means of staying fit. This may come as a letdown to those seeking an easy way to stay young and trim, but good health comes only through exercise that puts a stress on the heart, lungs and circulation. Massage is just too relaxing.

Good health comes down to three key factors: exercise, good food and plenty of sleep. First, exercise. Any number of sports will fit the bill, such as running, cycling, skiing (cross-country is superior to downhill in this category), racquetball, tennis, roller skating, and so on. All of these sports require the use of lungs and heart at a capacity that can be demanding. Don't expect to lose weight and become fit by riding around the block on your bicycle, coasting most of the way and eating a hot dog smothered in mustard. A vigorous and steady tempo is needed, something to get your heart pumping. The way to find out if you're working hard enough is to measure your heart beat. A simple formula says: take 220 and subtract your age. This is your maximum heart rate. To gain condition you must exercise to reach at least 60 to 70 percent of your maximum heart rate for about fifteen minutes, three to five days a week. To gain further insights on conditioning, read *Aerobics* by Kenneth Cooper or his more recent book *The New Aerobics*. Published in 1969 at the beginning of the health boom, *Aerobics* is still one of the most popular books on physical fitness, written for the person who has never been active. A point system rates the various sports according to their difficulty and tells you just how much time you need to spend at them to reach a reasonable fitness level. Cooper also presents a series of simple tests you can do at home to monitor what shape you're in before you begin the program of your choice.

Along with the good exercise plan, you need a sound diet. Diet does not refer to a weight-loss program, but the right food intake.

Exercising will take care of any weight concerns.

So much has been written about food, today's shoppers roam around the grocery store like lost souls. Does this hot dog have nitrites? Are these corn chips natural? Has this fruit been sprayed? You need to use common sense and weigh the good with the bad when it comes to choosing food. All food, no matter how "natural" has some kind of contamination. And a little chemical contamination won't hurt the human system. A lot will. You need to read between the lines of natural food hype and food industry brainwashing.

The most basic food diet has been around for decades and is still the most highly recommended by most nutritionists. They are speaking of the four basic food groups—meat (protein), dairy products, breads, and fruits and vegetables. A well-balanced diet includes some or all of these in three meals a day. If you eat something in each of the four food groups every day, there is nothing to fear in terms of vitamin deficiency, mineral deprivation or the like.

Avoid canned goods when you shop; rather, stick to the produce section and the meat department, but avoid red meats. Chicken and fresh fish are more easily digested and contain fewer additives. The more processing a product receives, the less nutritional value it will have. That means forego the mushy white bread for a solid loaf of whole wheat. That also goes for cooking; the more you cook the food, the more it will lose in vitamins and minerals.

Finally, sleep is the last link to good health and perhaps the best restorative mechanism for the human body. During sleep your heart beats at its lowest rate and tensions lessen; however, some people, even in sleep, have tight muscles and deep-seated anxieties that will reduce the quality of sleep. A massage before bed is a great way to lessen tensions built up over the day. But before receiving a massage you should give yourself at least two hours to digest your meal. A lot of blood is required to digest food and it is unwise to tax your system with a massage while blood is at work in the stomach. How much sleep do you need? The figure varies from person to person, but the common denominator is eight hours. Older people need less sleep, younger people need more, as do athletes in training. If you find yourself constantly tired during the day you may need more sleep or at least a higher quality.

6

Lotions and Potions

Massaging without oils would be like eating pumpkin pie minus the whipped cream or a chocolate chip cookie with no chocolate chips. Every massage practitioner relies on oils and would not work without them, unless, of course, the client requested otherwise. Some people do not like the feel of oil on their skin. But oils allow freer hand movement over the body, reduce friction and eliminate the pulling of body hairs. And oils have been around as long as massage.

The writings of Homer imply that, as early as 1000 B.C., an oily medium was used for massage. According to Homer's *Odyssey*, beautiful women rubbed and anointed the war-worn heroes to rest and refresh them. The story tells of Greek women also using oils, ". . . they all bathed in the sea, and anointed themselves with olive oil." Herodotus advised that a "greasy mixture" should be poured over the body before rubbing and Plato and Socrates refer in their writings to the benefit received from anointing with oils and rubbing as an "assuager of pain." Roman history records that the great orator Cicero enjoyed improved health because of his anointer.

Olive oil was the prime ingredient used in massage and was believed to have curative powers. The ancient belief about oils and lotions being good for the skin has survived the centuries, as witnessed by the many exotic lotions and creams made for women today. These lotions and creams have been marketed for a vast array of benefits—they soften and smooth your skin, they remove wrinkles overnight and make you more beautiful.

There is some truth that oils can help dry skin or skin in need of certain minerals, and natural healing herbs may be added to massage oils to be spread across the body. Check with your health food store for some of these herbs, which run the alphabetical gamut—aspen, armca, camphor, cajeput, caraway, elder, eucalyptus, juniper, lobeila, mace, marjoram, poke root, St. Johnswort, Soloman's Seal, tansy, witch hazel, wormwood. Their curative powers include antispasmodic, calmative, carminative, demulcent, diaphoretic, diuretic, nutritive and so on. It would take an entire book just to describe all these herbs and what they can do for you.

Numerous liniment ingredients include these herbs. Liniments are used on sore muscles, sprains, bruises and for general inflammation. They act as a counter-irritant to heat the skin and thus increase circulation to the affected area. They are especially popular with athletes who suffer from bruised muscles or painful joints. You might ask for a liniment rub at your next massage.

Dry massage was once quite popular and still has some adherents. They argue that it is cleaner, less messy and gives a certain feeling to the hand for steadier movements. But there is going to be more friction between the hand and the skin, as compared to oil, no matter how much talcum powder you use. Powders are recommended for absorbing moisture.

Commercial and mineral baby oils are not recommended for a full body massage, because, some practitioners argue, they are refined petroleum products devoid of vitamins. Some dermatologists maintain that they actually rob the body of vitamins upon entering the skin, although there is no evidence to confirm or deny this. The advantage mineral oils have over vegetable oils is that they are cheap and not subject to spoilage. In a pinch you can use a mineral oil but vegetable oil is so much more natural.

Vegetable oils have been in use by man for thousands of years, so they have a proven track record. Sweet almond oil mixed with smaller quantities of other oils and scented is currently popular. Coconut and olive oil are also popular, along with safflower and avocado. Other substances that can be used include glycerine, neat's-foot oil, fat, wool fat, petroleum jelly, lanolin, hog's lard, cold cream, peanut oil, cocoa butter, even sand. Yes, sand. Lotions work, too, but they are absorbed by the skin so quickly that frequent applications are required.

Almond oil is perhaps so popular now because of its characteristics; it is light in texture and scent and doesn't block the fragrance of herbs used with it. It is sensitive to heat, frying and turning rancid at lower temperatures than olive oil. You should store it in a glass container in a cool, dry place. When you're ready to give a massage, pour some of the oil into your squeeze bottle and heat it slowly in a pan of warm water. Applying cold oil to your partner will definitely result in a disagreeable reaction.

Whereas almond oil has been popular in the West, coconut oil is grounded in the Orient, where it is readily available. Coconut oil was extracted by mortar and pestle before more modern methods speeded up the process. Coconut oil also spoils easily so use caution when storing it.

When you think of olive oil you might imagine the sun-drenched hillsides of Italy with their row upon row of olive trees. Olive oil is one of the cheaper vegetable oils, unless you want to use the lowly corn oil, and has various quality grades. The clear, bland yellowish liquid is taken from the entire fruit, but the best quality is taken from the pulp. To obtain the finest oil, the fruit is picked by hand before it is fully ripened, peeled and subjected to gentle pressure without heat. Ripe fruit yields more oil, but of a less perfect flavor. Recently, it has been altered by the addition of other oils, such as cottonseed and sesame, but laws now require that it be labeled salad oil if it contains any foreign ingredients.

Many of these oils are available at the grocery store in large-quantity packaging that can offer substantial savings. The most expensive way to purchase an oil for massage is to buy it in the health food store or from a massage studio that prepackages it; If you'll read the contents label you'll see that there are no magic formulas, just good, old-fashioned vegetable oil and some nice scents.

Glycerin is not used for massage alone, but is sometimes mixed with an oil base because it is valuable as a moistener, by absorbing water from the air. The colorless, odorless, sweet-tasting syrupy liquid is composed of carbon, hydrogen and oxygen. It is obtained from fats as a by-product in the manufacture of soaps and fatty acids or it can be synthesized commercially from propylene. It is used in many women's cosmetics.

Believe it or not, lanolin, the grease from wool, is an excellent skin conditioner and is used in many lip balm preparations. The greasy, yellow substance is a chemical mixture of cholesterol and the esters of several fatty acids. With water it forms an emulsion. You may find it in some massage centers.

Isopropyl alcohol is sometimes used in massage when mixed with water. However, it evaporates quickly and cools the skin. Most people don't like the cooling effect, but on a hot day it might be a great solution for beating the heat. Alcohol is also used after a massage to help remove oil.

Whatever oil you use, you will be able to scent it with an essence extract, a perfume or a few drops of fresh lemon juice. The scent you create can set the mood of a massage.

There is no perfect technique for using oil on your partner and with time you will develop a keen sense of knowing when it is time to add oil. On parts of the body with considerable hair you will need to apply a little more oil. Other body parts such as the ear and face will need little, if any. People with dry skin need more oil than people with oily skin. Before you begin stroking, apply the oil liberally to your hands and to your forearms if you intend to use them for massage.

7

Learning the Techniques

Hands are the tools of the masseur's or masseuse's trade, and wondrous instruments they are. A man-made machine has yet to duplicate their amazing dexterity, nor can any known drug reproduce their ability to bring comfort and relaxation. Your hands go about bringing happiness to someone through massage, in which there are five major motions—friction, stroking (effleurage), kneading (petrissage), percussion (tapotement) and vibration. You can use the palms of your hands, your fingers or your thumbs, one hand or two, your wrists, even your forearm to massage. No matter how many techniques or how much practical theory you know, however, you must develop the right touch. With time you will learn just how much pressure to place on various parts of the body, what areas respond best to a particular technique and how many strokes you should give or how long to apply friction.

Whatever technique you employ, it is important to remember some of the fundamentals: 1) make smooth transitions between parts of the body; 2) keep your fingernails short and well-trimmed; 3) whenever your partner expresses the slightest hint of pain, back off (unless it has been established before the massage begins that pain, e.g., from working knots out of tight muscles, is acceptable); 4) never lose contact with your partner; 5) work at a steady pace and with confidence; 6) when you begin the massage, say with the head, work your way downward in a logical manner—to the neck, then the arms, the chest, the hips and so on; 7) work one side of the body completely before having your partner turn over.

Pain experienced during massage can indicate several different problems; you might be kneading too hard, your partner might have a tender muscle where there is pain or your technique is being improperly administered. If relaxation is your aim, be sure to have your partner tell you when he experiences pain. But there are occasions when pain is unavoidable, for instance, when you have found a knot of muscles in need of loosening. The only way to free them is by applying considerable pressure.

Certain parts of the body are obviously more sensitive to pain than others. Use caution when working the eyes, ears and toes. On the other hand, you can really bare down on the back and the appendages, where the muscles are broad and strong.

Losing physical contact with your partner brings a different sort of pain—the emotional pain of uncertainty. It puts your partner's nerves on the alert and leads to bad vibrations. It leaves him wondering, "Where will I be touched next?" In addition to maintaining contact, your movements should be sure. To avoid hesitation, think ahead about where your hands will go and what part of the body you will concentrate on next. If you're just learning, an understanding partner, perhaps a close friend, can help instill confidence through encouragement. At the same time they'll allow you to make mistakes without fear of reprimand.

The following techniques are commonplace in Esalen and Swedish massage and each has its own value in stimulating the body and its most appropriate location for application.

FRICTION

How it's done. Friction incorporates the fingertips, thumbs, heel of the hand or the dorsal surface of the two terminal phalanges. The whole or part of the hand is moved over the surface with a good degree of pressure, the amount varying in different parts—heavy over thick, fleshy skin and light over bony surfaces or thin tissues. Pressure should not be so great that the hand will not readily slide over the surface or interfere with the movement of the blood in the arteries. Pressure should be applied before moving your hand and always should be toward a bony support. Keep your fingers elastic and try to use the muscles of your upper arm and shoulder to reduce stress on your hands, which will otherwise tire easily. Start the friction gently and increase pressure gradually, moving your hand back and forth.

Where to do it. Friction feels good just about anywhere you use it. It aids in the removal of inflammation, increases circulation, loosens adherent scars and stretches contracted muscles. Working in circles with your hands you can massage the stomach to increase blood flow, which quickens digestion. Go clockwise. If your partner has tendinitis, friction is particularly effective in reducing the pain and speeding recovery. There are two kinds of friction: centripetal friction is movement in the direction of the venous blood flow and by far the most common. Centrifugal friction is movement opposite to venous blood flow. In other words, downward friction decreases vascular activity.

STROKING (EFFLEURAGE)

How it is done. Stroking is simply touch combined with motion. It is the most basic and most often used massage method and the easiest to learn. All you do is lightly move the tips of two, three or all of your fingers, or your entire hand or both hands, gently over your partner's body. Gentle stroking, which is great for inducing relaxation, calls for less than the full weight of your hand resting on your partner. The wrist must be kept flexible and the movement even, slow and uniform in relation to pressure and time. It will require some practice to get the feel for the right movement but once you've got the hang of it your sixth sense will tell you that your partner is fully enjoying the massage.

Relax your hand while stroking. Frigid hands or fingers feel like lava rocks rubbing soft flesh and the enjoyment of the massage is lost. Instead, control motion through the muscles of the upper body and arm, once again, so that your hands will not take the burden of the exercise. Move from the outside to the center of the area being worked. Stroke at least three times on a given area, moving at the rate of about one or two inches a second. Stroking may be repeated at the same place until the desired effect is produced. This may lead you to stroke the leg, for example, dozens of times, gradually increasing the pressure and the speed of movement as you go.

Remember, stroking is in only one direction and if you move back and forth you're inducing friction. The direction of deep stroking is normally with the venous flow, while light stroking can be against the venous flow.

Where to do it. Wherever your hands can reach, stroking is appropriate. Stroking is uniquely effective for the nervous system. A light stroke with two fingers tracing the edges of your partner's spine stimulates the nervous system and feels good. Sometimes stroking becomes so relaxing that your partner goes to sleep during the massage. Should this happen, continue working and he'll probably sleep right through it.

KNEADING (PETRISSAGE)

How it is done. This is perhaps the most complex of the massage techniques, with its many variations. Basically, kneading is the grasping of your partner's skin with your hands and intermittent compression against the underlying bony surface. Your partner's muscles are grasped between the fingers and thumb, lifted from the bone and squeezed. The grasp is then relaxed and by a movement of the wrist, without losing contact with the limb, a fresh grasp is taken immediately below the first and the movement is repeated. Pressure should always be applied in an upward direction and in line with the bone. Don't twist the muscle.

On large surfaces the hands (or hand) are pressed down and moved in a circular motion, causing compression of soft parts of the harder structures. Pressure should be applied in a wave-like manner to get alternate compression and relaxation. When kneading the limbs, which is one of the best places to work using this procedure, you should grasp the muscle being worked with your entire hand, lifting alternately and squeezing and relaxing it while moving it in a circular motion.

There are two variations of kneading—deep and superficial. Deep kneading is the best-known form; the muscles are grabbed like a lump of clay, using as much of your hand as possible, and pulled outward from the bone, stretching the underlying tissue. Superficial kneading is like pinching and affects just the skin and surface nerves. The skin is simultaneously pressed between the thumb and finger and lifted from the underlying bone or muscle, being released at the moment when strain is the greatest. This gives the maximum effect in emptying and refilling the blood vessels and lymph spaces and channels.

Another form of kneading is rolling. In this system the tissues of your partner are compressed against the bone and rolled by a to-and-fro movement. In rolling, the fingers are extended and held closely together. You can use one or both hands and the movement is a quick one, between 200 and 400 strokes a minute, and with considerable pressure. Imagine rolling as taking a thick wad of clay and rubbing it between your hands until it gets thin and long.

Lastly, there is wringing. Grasp a limb with two hands, placed on opposite sides and close together. Then begin twisting movements with your hands, either simultaneously in the same direction or in alternation. If alternate movements are used, your hands must be separated a little. This is best done on the arms and legs and is a slow movement, around thirty strokes per minute.

Where to do it. Much of kneading is restricted to the limbs or fleshy surfaces, where there is a readily graspable mass of tissue with a strong undersurface, like bone. It is also best done on the limbs because the hands can completely encircle them, which is necessary for the rolling or wringing movement.

PERCUSSION (TAPOTEMENT)

How it is done. This is one of the more physically active movements, commonly associated with Swedish massage, although it is done with Esalen, too. The wrists and hands stroke quickly and lightly on the body. There are four types: clapping, hacking, tapping and beating. While this may sound like it could be a harmful activity, these movements are certainly not meant to cause pain; they are most pleasurable if done properly. Percussion's notoriety goes all the way back to the ancient Turkish baths and was popular, according to author Heinrich Wolf, *Textbook of Physical Therapy*, because its action made the people think they were really being treated, although Wolf argues that it has received far more attention than it deserves.

Whether or not you believe in percussion for treatment, the movements are given here just in case your masseur uses it or you choose to employ it: Clapping—using the entire hand, the palmar surface is shaped so as to entrap the air as it comes into contact with the skin, producing a sound not unlike clapping two hands together. Hacking—turn your hand on edge, using the ulnar or little finger and the border of the hand only. Hold the fingers lightly apart or loosely so that they are made to come successively in contact by the force of the blow, thus giving a peculiar vibratory effect. Tapping—extend the fingers in a rigid manner and use the palmar surfaces, keeping a rapid rhythm. Beating—strike the body with the palmar surface of a half-closed fist, the dorsal surface of the terminal phalanges of the fingers and the heel of the hand when coming in contact with the skin. Beating is a slow movement. Your relaxed arm is lifted from the shoulder, and then allowed to fall by its own weight. Pounding—with a quick movement use the ulnar border of the loosely closed hand by means of flexion and extensions of the elbow.

Where to use it. The location you choose for percussion depends on the particular style you employ, although its use is not recommended on delicate or sensitive parts of the body. Clapping is most effective on fleshy parts where strong surface stimulation is desired. It also works well on the chest for improving the interchange of gases and in loosening mucous. Hacking can be done on the chest, spine and the head. When you use percussion just remember not to hurt your partner. To avoid bruising, the arms and hands should not be held stiffly while making contact.

VIBRATION

How it is done. Vibration can be soothing or stimulatory, depending on how it is done. To give a soothing motion, relax your flat hand lightly on your partner. Rapidly contract and relax the forearm for the movement. To stimulate, use the fingertips, keeping them stationary on your partner. You might want to run your fingers down a nerve for stimulation of a large area.

Where to use it. Vibration is especially successful on fleshy areas, such as the stomach and the posterior. A unique and relaxing movement using vibration and recommended by George Downing in *The Massage Book* calls for vibration of the posterior. He says that you should place the butt of your hand on your partner's posterior with fingers outstretched like a fan. Then begin rapidly vibrating your hand on the fleshy posterior for a soothing sensation. Deep vibration can be used over an organ to give it direct stimulation, as well.

8

Laying of the Hands

PREPARATIONS

Before beginning the massage be sure that the setting is agreeable to both parties. What may be acceptable to you may not be to someone else. Consider the degree of privacy you desire. If you want to conduct a massage outside don't be surprised when hikers spot the two of you or when a plane flies overhead and begins circling. Indoors, choose a quiet location and disconnect nearby telephones.

Crucial to the professional massage is communication between client and practitioner. Practitioners, while they can do great things for sore, tight muscles, cannot read minds. Tell the practitioner—before the massage—just what you want done. Some suggestions for specific requests include 1) style of massage; 2) the pace, fast or slow; 3) amount of conversation between yourself and the practitioner; 4) music—if so, type—or no music; 5) where to begin and end, if you have a preference; 6) indicating areas that are tender to the touch or extremely sensitive; 7) giving a brief history of your health; 8) amount of pressure you desire during the effleurage stroking; 9) cost of the massage.

Proper room temperature is crucial to enjoying the massage. If it is less than 75 degrees Fahrenheit, your partner will likely become chilled. Once the massage begins, you and the practitioner may notice a slight increase in body temperature as circulation, from giving and receiving the massage, is stimulated. Taking a hot shower prior to the massage will not only relax you, but increase your body temperature as well.

A nude massage is not a requirement. Should your practitioner insist you remove all of your clothing and you are uncomfortable with that, consider taking your business elsewhere. Some people, for whatever reason, feel uncomfortable being unclothed with someone they are unfamiliar with, in anything but a medical setting, and even then they may not be fully comfortable. There are enough emotional concerns to deal with during your first massage without having to worry about nudity. Your practitioner should show some compassion and understanding and encourage you to wear what you please. Of course, not many practitioners are going to give massage to someone who is fully dressed. A good compromise is draping. The practitioner uses a towel or blanket to cover a client's body everywhere but the location being massaged. It may take a couple of massage sessions before you are comfortable with the idea that nudity does not equal sex: once you are comfortable, a nude massage will not only be acceptable, but the only way to go.

Proper lighting adds considerably to the soothing atmosphere of a massage; improper lighting can cause eye strain and tight muscles. Avoid bright, overhead lights. Lying on a table and looking up at bright lights is an uncomfortable experience; it may remind you of the hospital operating table or of being interrogated by space invaders while held captive on their flying saucer. Overhead lights tense eye muscles, which contributes to tight body muscles elsewhere. Use indirect or shaded light. Candlelight is a nice touch. In this atmosphere the scent of burning incense completes the mood.

If you have a professional massage, chances are it will be given on a massage table. That's because a practitioner can stand upright during the massage and thus reduce the need to bend his back, as would be required if the massage were given on the floor. A table also makes it easier for the practitioner to reach every part of your body, because it is somewhat narrow. A friendly at-home massage can be done on the floor, with a mat or sleeping bag used for padding, or on a picnic table with a foam pad. Don't use a soft bed, because it is hard to work all the body and beds are usually too wide to be convenient for the person giving the massage.

You may even decide to purchase a massage table, which involves a considerable investment and some brands are of questionable quality. Your local massage center can provide the best brand

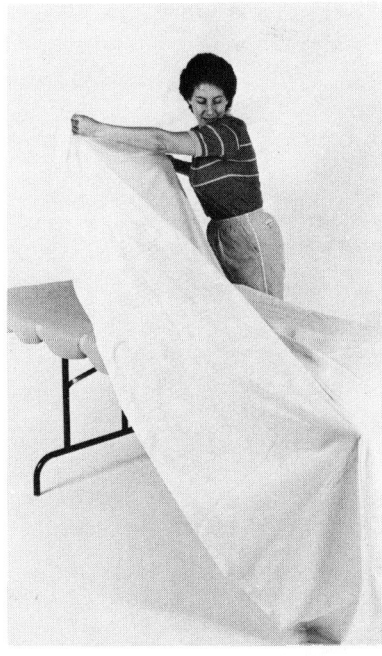

A table enables the practitioner to have more leverage. Any narrow table with the right "height" will do. Just be sure it has some padding.

names or you can even build your own, from instructions given in *The New Massage*, by Gordon Inkeles or *The Massage Book*, by George Downing.

Music and massage are complementary, although there are those who prefer silence during the massage in order to heighten the experience. Most massage centers offer music, always mellow and melodic. Ask for it before the massage begins.

Most practitioners use a squeeze bottle for holding massage oil; however, some prefer an open bowl, into which they dip their hands or fingers. Squeeze bottles won't spill oil all over the new carpet when dropped and are more convenient to use. For more on oils and their affect, see Chapter 4.

Finally, be sure that you have removed all jewelry, watches, glasses, earrings, hearing aids and contact lenses—before the massage begins. Contact lenses are so non-intrusive that they are often forgotten. But the eyes cannot be safely massaged if contact lenses are worn. If you have left the lenses on, tell the practitioner, and if you have forgotten to remove some jewelry (or can't get it off) the practitioner can work around it or take it off for you.

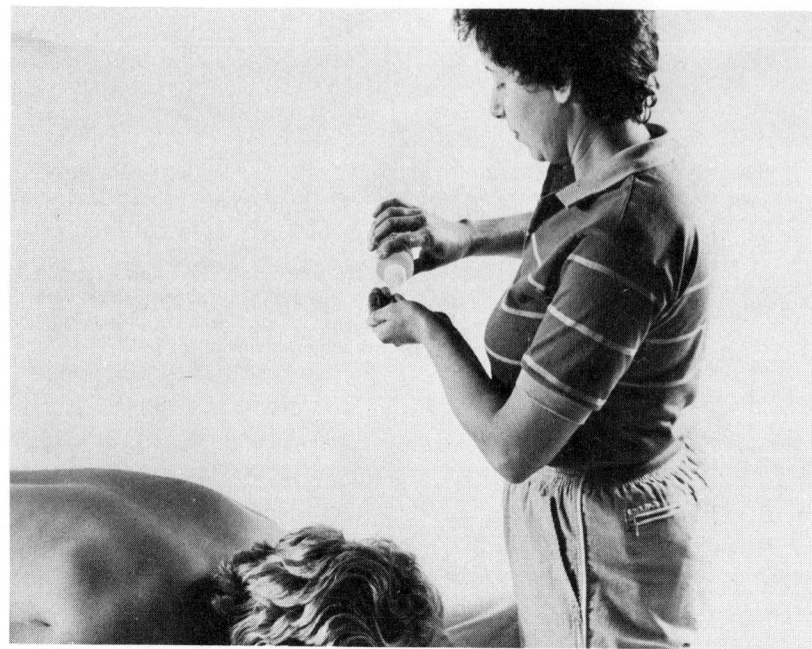

Squeeze bottles are handy to use and won't spill the oil.

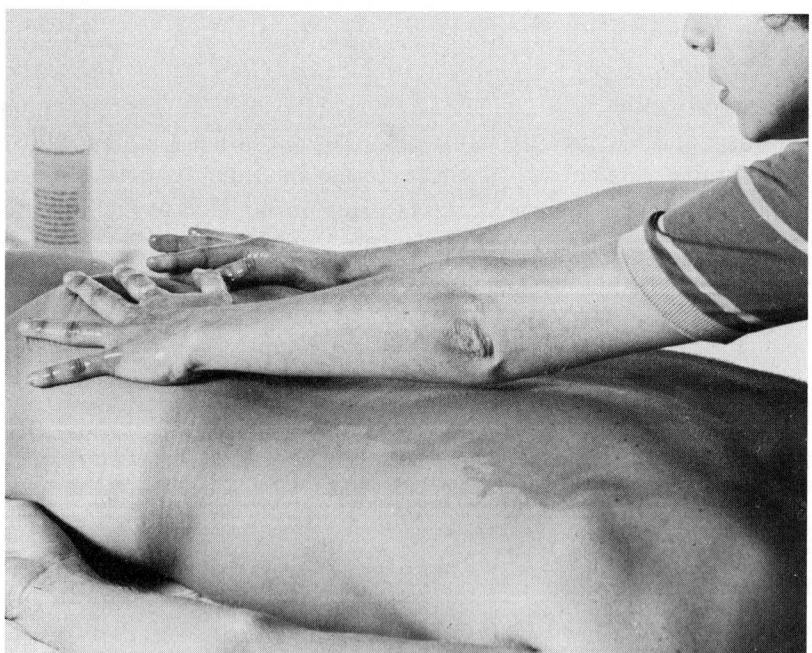

Before beginning the massage, oil down your partner.

STEP-BY-STEP

The following massage procedure has been described by Robin Tobias, a physical therapist at the Sunnyvale Physical Therapy and Sports Injury Center, in Sunnyvale, California, who is certified in massage and Trager bodywork, and Linda Chrisman, a partner of The Massage Center in Palo Alto, and certified in massage and Trager bodywork. Their techniques have been developed over the years to include Swedish and Esalen styles of relaxation and enjoyment. In addition, they like to include gentle stretching movements during the massage. The massage techniques you will read here are basic and you will probably recognize many of them, should you receive a professional massage. Of course, there are literally thousands of variations to these movements and you can explore with a friend to discover and enjoy them. Realize, too, that personal taste enters into the experience, both for the practitioner and the client.

The first rule for the person massaging is to clear any thoughts he* might have about his own problems and to try to detach himself so that the time spent in the session is the client's, not the practitioner's. Your partner will probably want to lie on his stomach to begin. That position exposes the back, our least vulnerable side and the area that most people feel comfortable exposing first. Many of us also carry a lot of tension in our backs and to work there first will help reduce some of that tension level, making the rest of the massage easier. Lying on the stomach, however, can be stressful to his neck, so when your partner turns over you should massage his neck. Also, ask him to turn his head occasionally during the massage when he is on his stomach.

BODY STROKES

In order to simplify the descriptions that follow, we will define particular strokes used often. They are:
● **Circle Eight**—Place both hands on your partner, side by side with thumbs touching. Move the left hand in a small clockwise

*The word "he" is used to describe the partner throughout this chapter (and generally in the complete text) as a matter of clarity and convenience. Obviously, massage enjoyment is not restricted to the male species. And, the word practitioner has been used to describe the masseur or masseuse whenever possible.

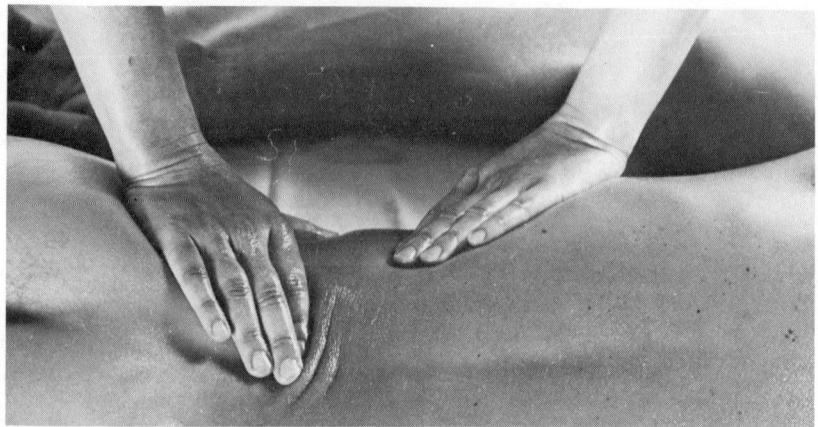

Start the circle-eight stroke with both hands on your partner.

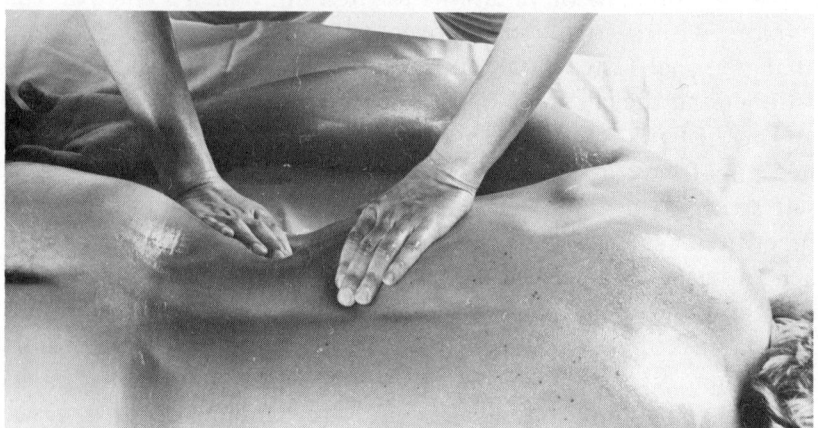

Move the left hand in a small clockwise circle.

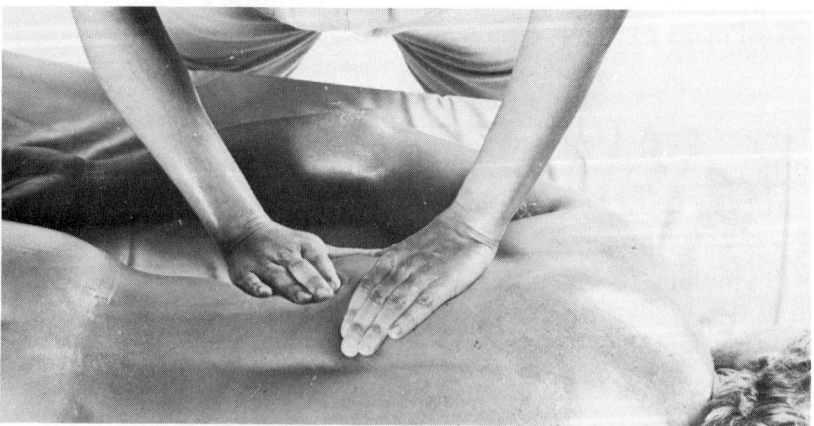

Move your right hand in a clockwise circle when your left hand completes a circle.

circle. Return it to make a full circle, then move your other hand, also clockwise, to complete the other half of the figure-eight. Repeat this rhythmic movement of both hands as you move across the body.

● **V-stroke**—Keeping your fingers together, spread your thumb to form a v-shape. You may use one hand or both hands.

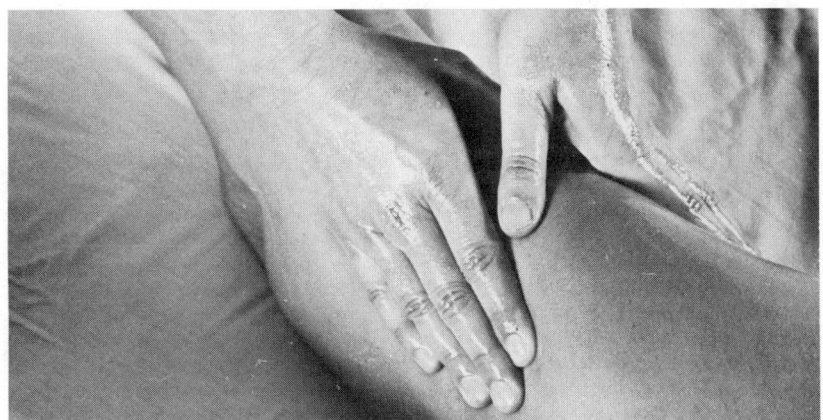

Separate your thumb from your fingers for the V-stroke.

● **Hand-Over-Hand**—Begin with both hands on your partner, one in front of the other. Now bring the hand closest to you back toward your body. You will lift it off the body to complete that

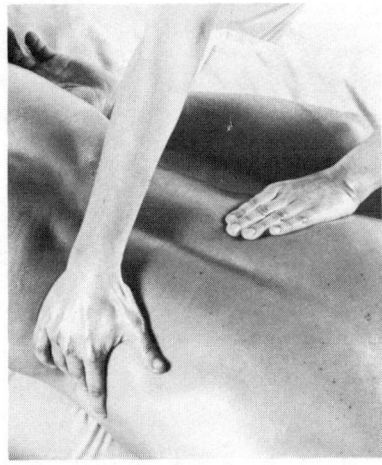

Right hand is placed on side of the body in hand-over-hand stroke

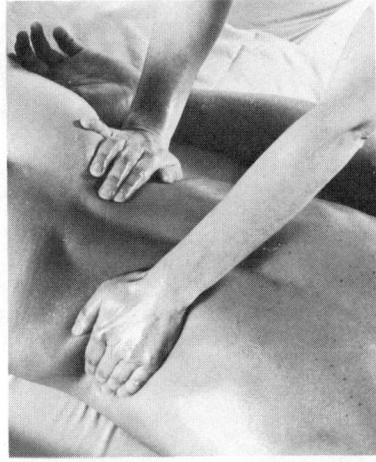

Now right hand moves to same position left hand occupied.

part of the stroke. As you bring your hand through the air to where you started the stroke, pull the front hand back across the same area the other hand just covered. Continue this "petting" motion using both hands.

● **Push-Pull**—Place both hands side by side on your partner. Push one hand away while pulling the other toward you, slightly lifting the musculature and letting it sink back down.

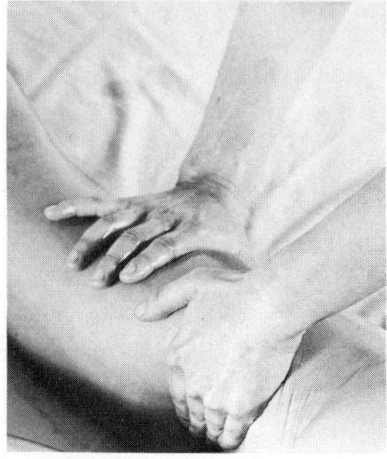
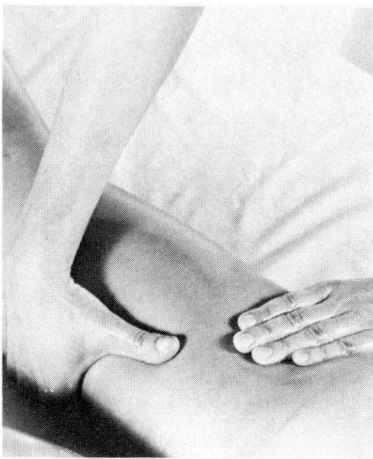

Left hand pulls and right hand pushes in this push-pull stroke.

Now left hand is pushing, right hand pulling.

● **Pulling**—Using both hands simultaneously or one hand at a time, pull on the body, hands moving toward your body on the

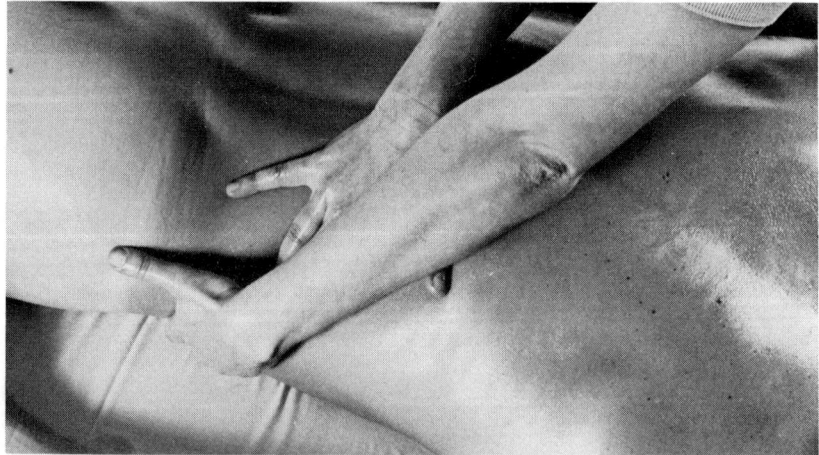

The pulling stroke as shown on the back.

return stroke. Usually this movement is done with hands perpendicular to the long axis of the body.

Other more general massage techniques such as effleurage, petrissage, kneading and friction are described in Chapter 7.

BACK

To start, stand in front of your partner's head. Place both hands on your partner's shoulders, fingers spread and pointed toward his feet. If you are working on the floor, straddle your partner's head between your thighs. Most of your back strokes will be down toward your partner's toes; this runs contrary to the physiological rule-of-thumb that tells us to stroke toward the heart, but venous flow is not the only concern in sensual massage.

Begin with an effleurage (French for "to flow") stroke, using light hand strokes that should gradually increase in pressure. Push your hands down both sides of your partner's spine as you lean forward, using your body weight to exert pressure. Stroke down over the buttocks, around the gluteal fold and then return up the sides of the back. Now bring your hands onto the shoulder and then over the back of the arms (halfway to the elbow). Finish the stroke where your hands started on the back.

Don't stroke the spine itself when your hands are moving down your partner's back. Repeat this movement three or four times and by the last stroke you should be exerting the deepest pressure.

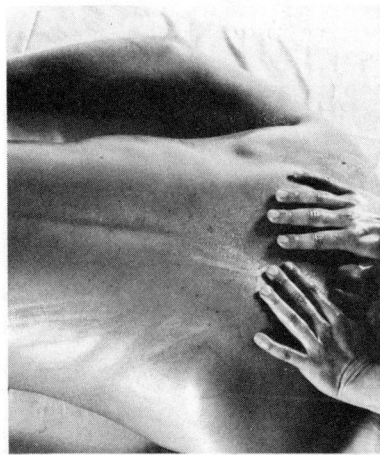

A complete back stroke begins at the shoulders.

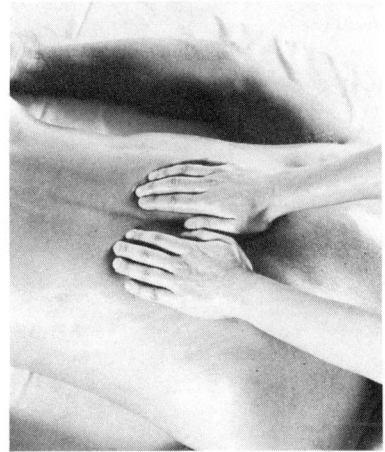

Use the effleurage stroke.

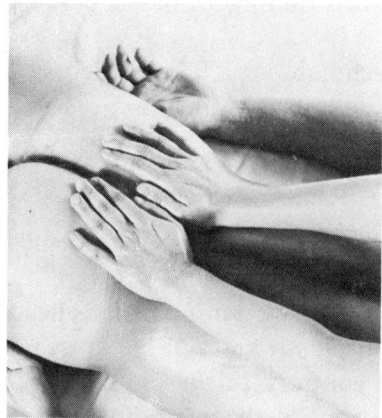

Use your body weight to exert pressure.

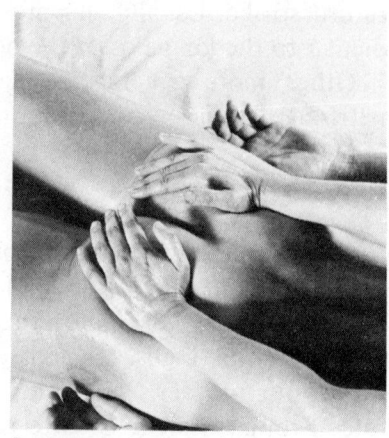

Stroke over the glueteal fold.

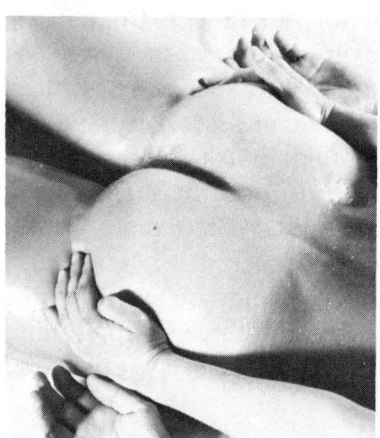

Begin the return stroke.

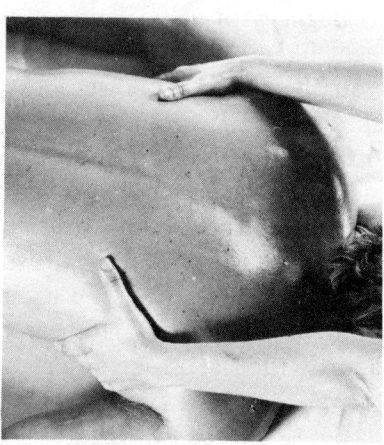

Separate hands and move up sides of body.

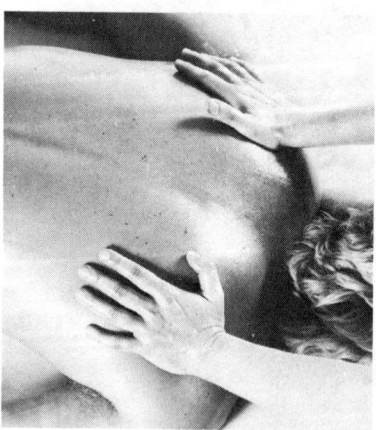

You're back where you started.

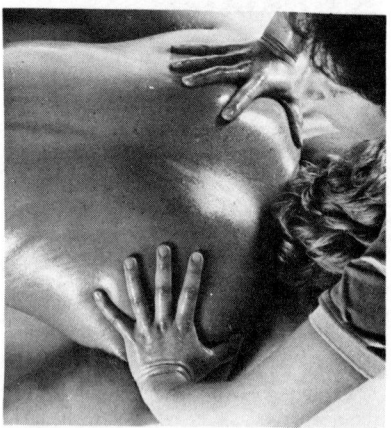

Spread hands again and move over shoulders.

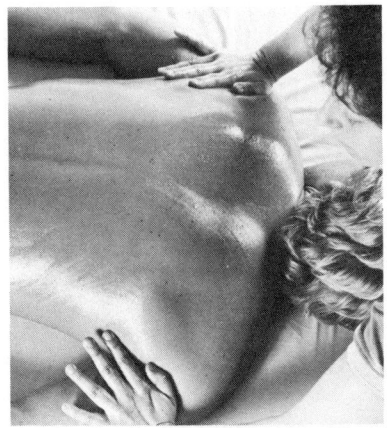

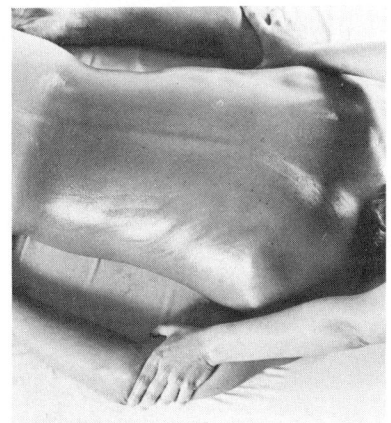

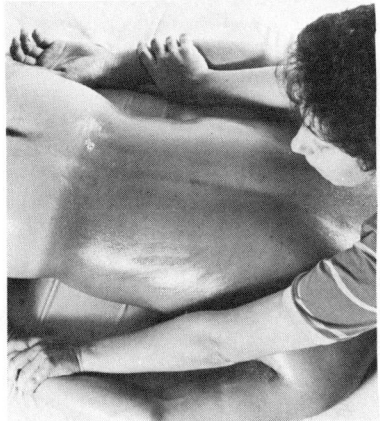

Stroke down both arms. Use a smooth, flowing motion. You may finish at the hands.

Now stand on one side, facing away from your partner. Use the hand-over-hand effleurage stroke. Begin at the shoulder nearest you and travel down one side of the back to the gluteals, continuing over the buttocks and down the leg. You may increase pressure on the posterior because this is a fleshy area with plenty of padding. Your fingers should be spread and relaxed, following the contours of the body as they point toward your partner's feet. Add oil during this full body stroke as needed, to achieve a smooth, gliding motion. Move down to the heel of the foot and then over the arch and toes, finishing here. When you stroke the feet during the full body stroke be sure to use considerable pressure to avoid tickling. Stroke the foot using hand-over-hand effleurage several more times.

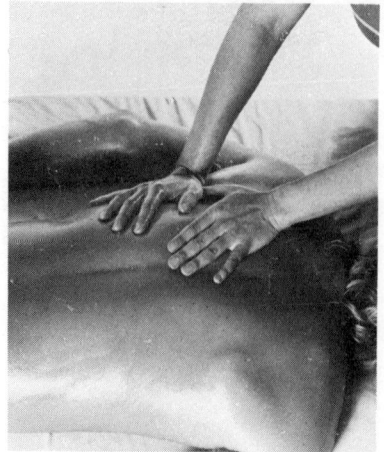

Now stroke down one side of the back.

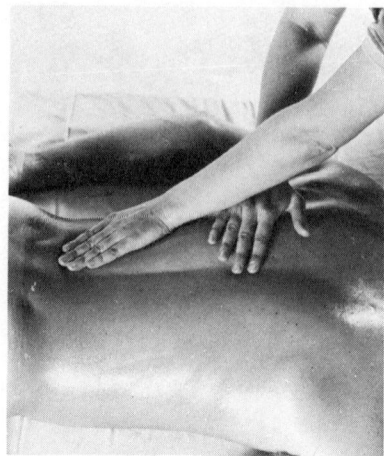

Use the hand-over-hand effleurage stroke.

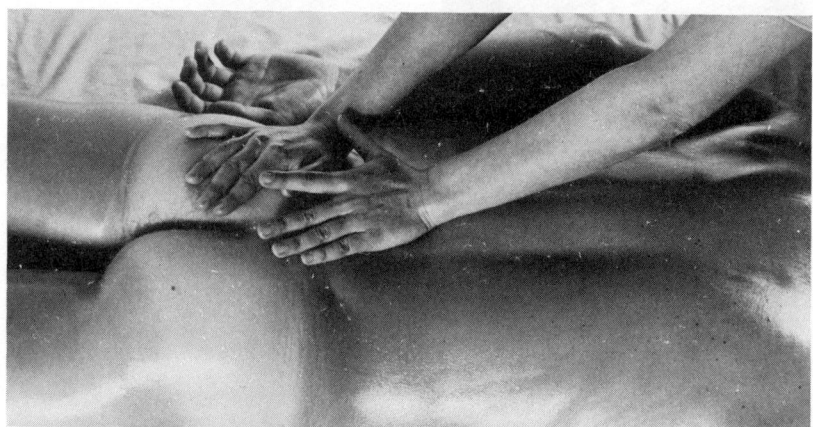

Increase pressure on the posterior.

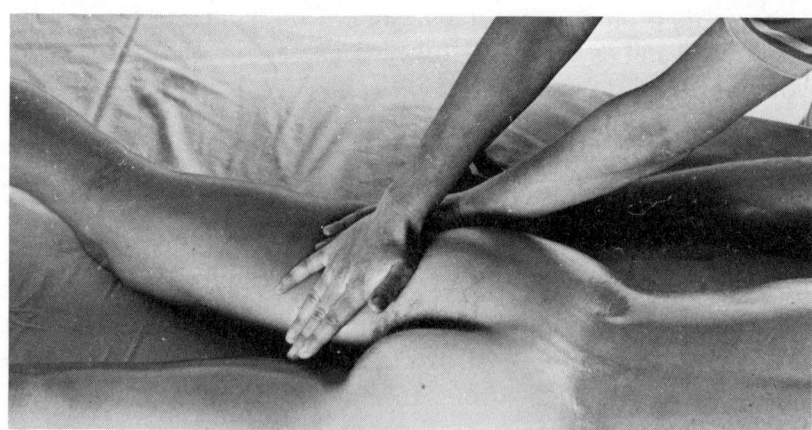

Your fingers should be spread and relaxed.

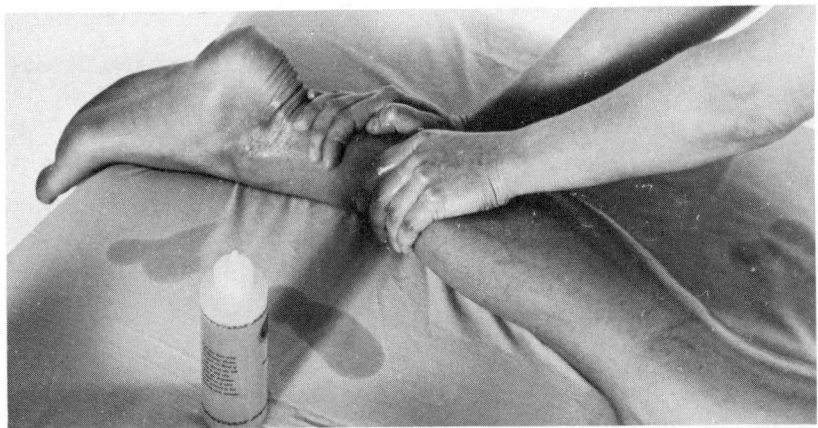

Stroke the length of the calf muscle.

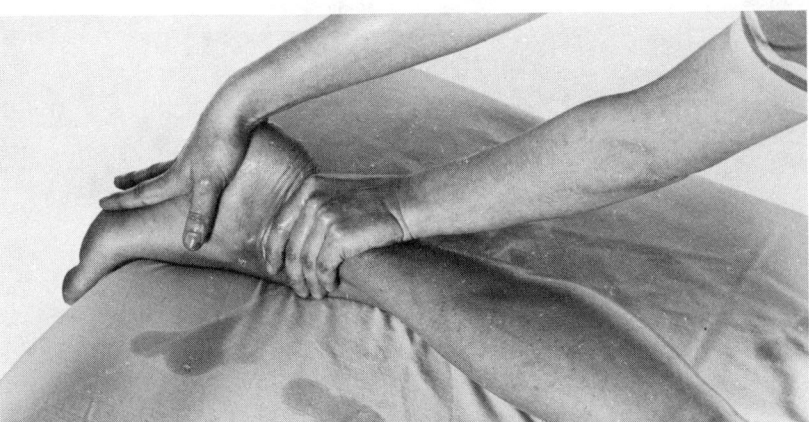

Finish the stroke at the foot.

The return stroke is slightly different. Wrap both hands around your partner's ankle, one hand in front of the other. Now simultaneously bring both hands back toward the shoulder while retracing your previous stroke. You can repeat this on the other side.

Here is a stretch for the back muscles. Stand at your partner's side. Begin with both hands resting next to one another, fingers pointing toward and perpendicular to the spine, in the middle of one side of your partner's back. Now simultaneously spread your hands and arms apart, one hand moving toward your partner's buttocks and the other moving up toward his neck. Besides stretching the back, this movement gives a feeling of length and

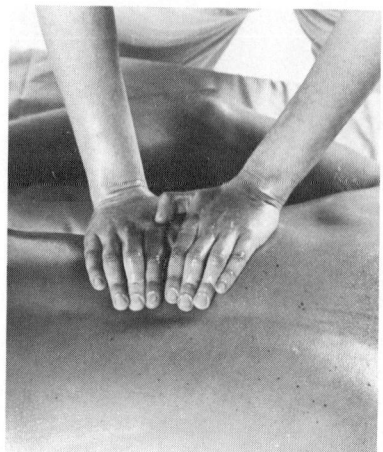

This is a good stroke to stretch back muscles.

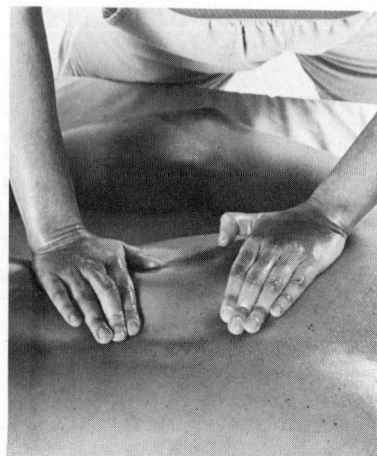

Keep your hands perpendicular to the spine.

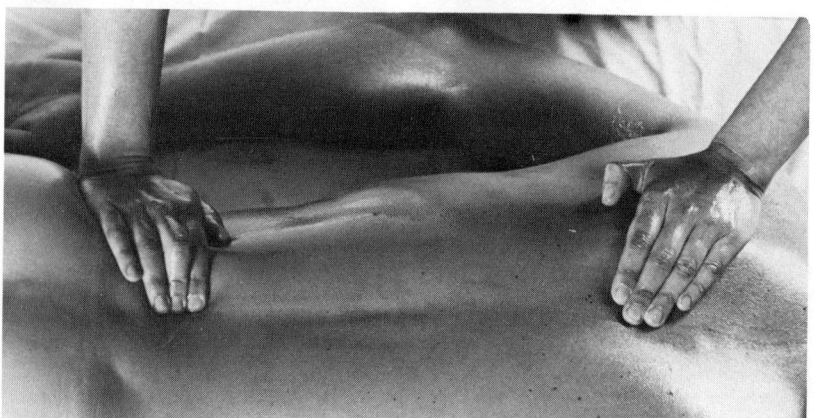

Move your hands apart, exerting pressure.

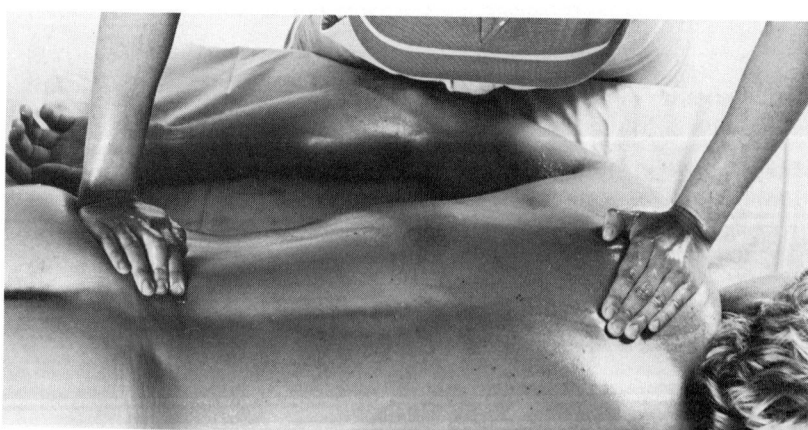

Finish with hands at the gluteal fold and on back of the neck.

unity to your partner. Stretch the other side of the back after moving to the other side of the table.

This massage stroke calls for circular motions. Begin at the base of the neck and make deep, slow circles (not friction, but close) with your thumbs. Run the thumbs down both sides of the spine, to the sacral region, on both sides. Use your fingers to lead your

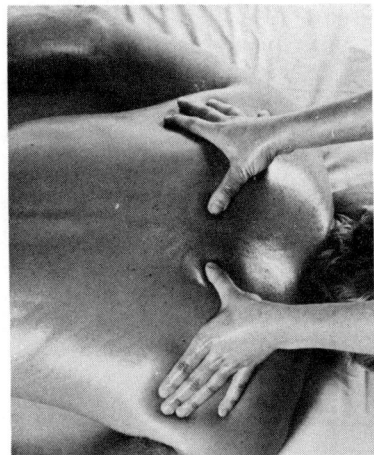

Begin stroke for paraspinal muscles with hands on each side of the spine.

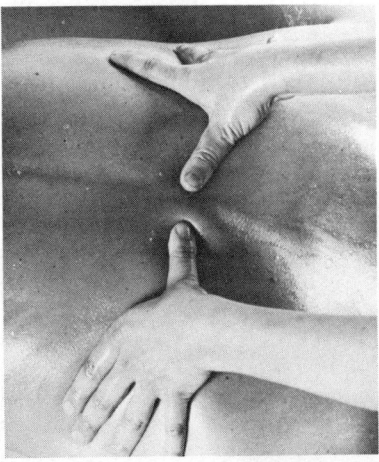

Trace the edge of the spine with your thumbs.

Keep your thumbs off the spine itself.

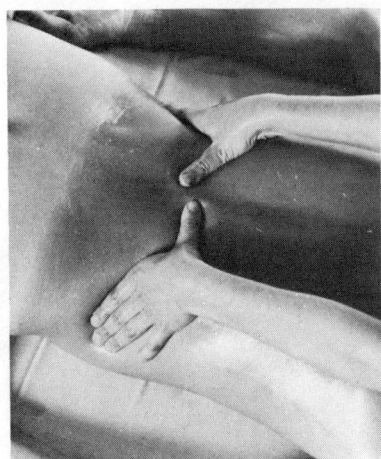

Return after reaching the lower back.

thumb, but don't exert pressure with them. This stroke works the paraspinal muscles. They are long, thin muscles that extend from the sacrum to the neck, on either side of the spine.

Keep your body behind your hands for increased leverage and to allow yourself the maximum rest when stroking the back. (Also, the table height is important if you want to avoid back strain. Here is how to determine the proper table height for you: extend your arm at your side, bending your hand at the wrist so that the palm of your hand is parallel with the floor. The palm of your hand should be level with the table top or slightly higher.)

Next we move to the pulling stroke. Stand at your partner's side. Begin by placing your hands on your partner's side farthest from you, reaching across the table. From the hip, work up to your partner's armpit, pulling toward the spine. The movement creates a lifting sensation. Use your fingers to grasp and your body to pull. To work the side of the body nearest you, shift around to

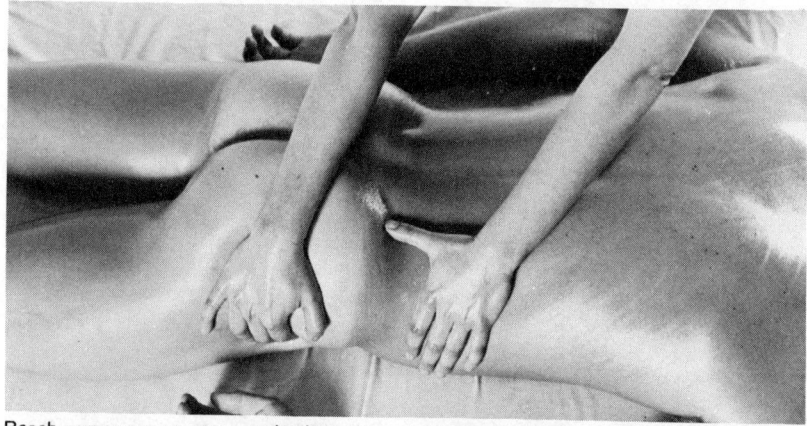

Reach across your partner to do the pulling stroke on the back.

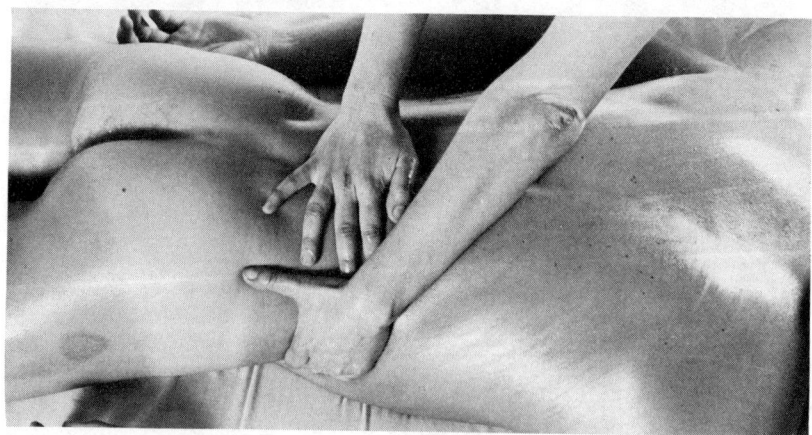

Start at the hip and work up to the armpit.

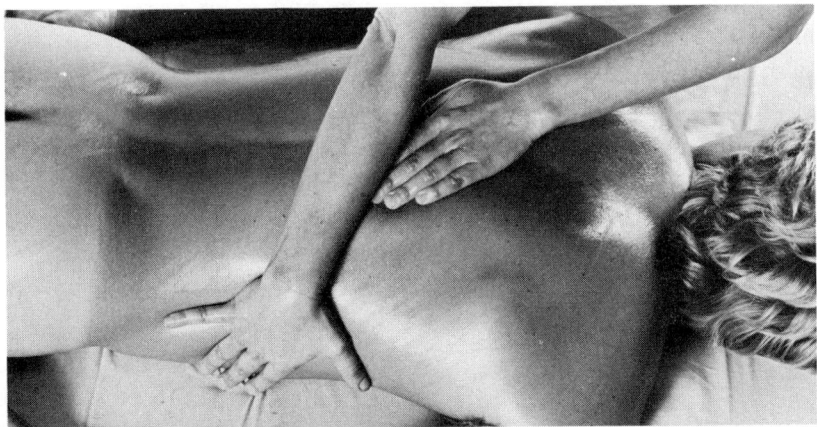

Your partner will feel a "lifting" sensation.

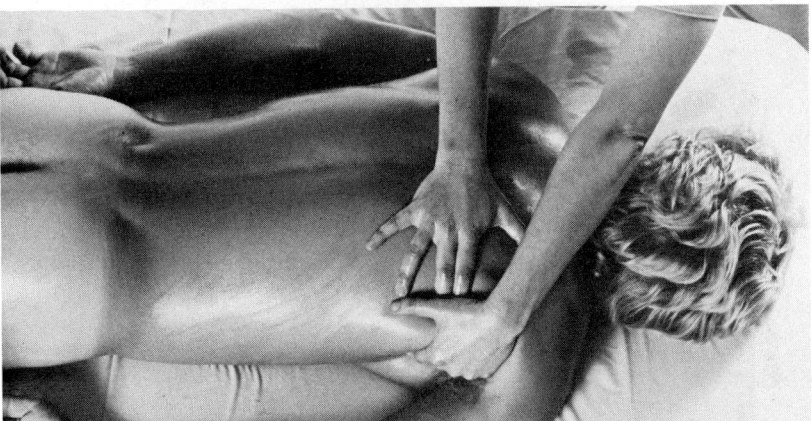

You can alternate hands while stroking.

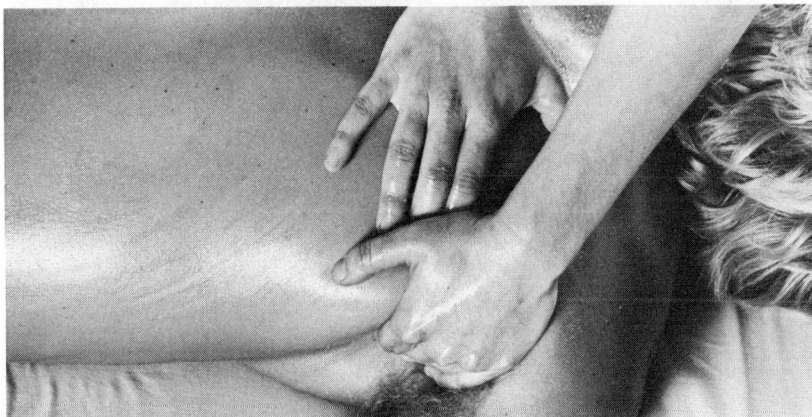

Put your hand close to the armpit.

the opposite side of your partner and pull from there. Or, you may want to push up against the side, stroking from your partner's side up to his back. The heel of one hand begins at the side of your partner and pushes up toward the spine.

A circle-eight stroke is also recommended for the back. Start in the lumbo-sacral area and spread your fingers and thumb apart to form a v-shape. Work up to the scapula, where there usually isn't enough muscle tissue to pick up.

Now work the trapezius. Stand at your partner's side, by his shoulder, facing him. Keeping your hands in a v-shape, move

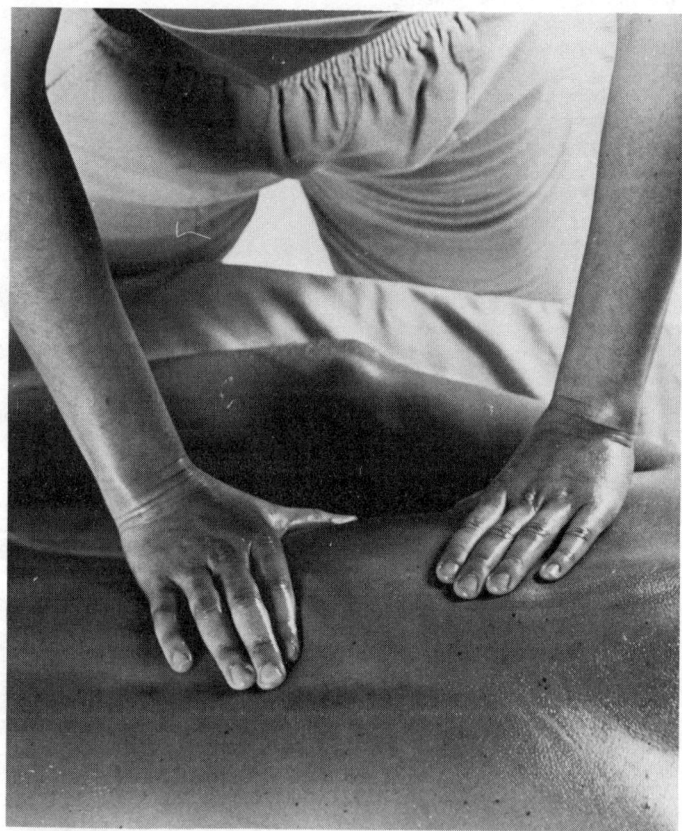

A circle-eight stroke starting on the lower back.

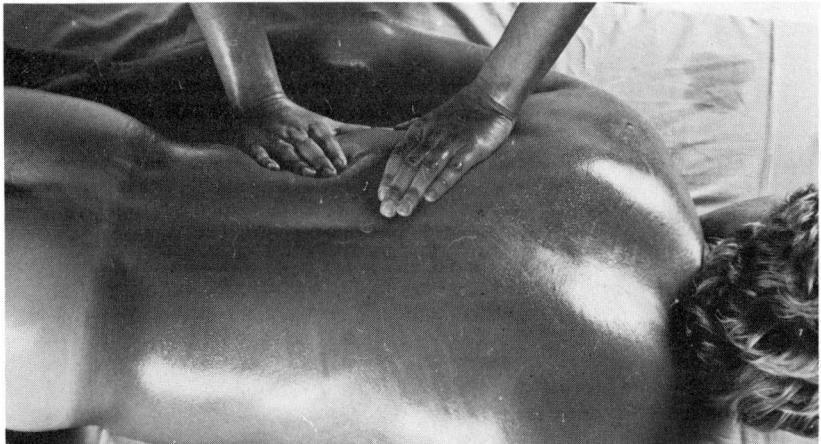

Work up the back toward the shoulder.

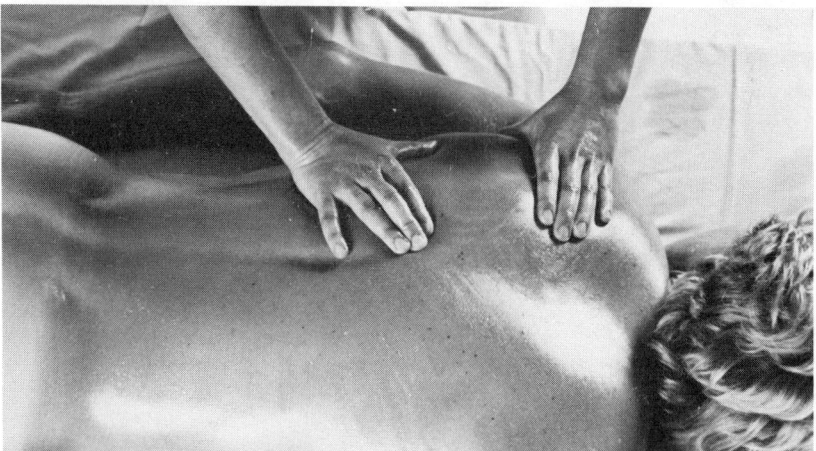

Form a v-shape with your hands.

one hand over and down the trapezius, using the thumb of your other hand to trace the medial border of the scapula. This hand can be spread and used to stroke the back.

For people who work hunched over a desk all day, here is a good massage technique for their sore rhomboid (both major and minor) muscles. These muscles attach to the upper back in the spine and extend over to the scapula, pulling the scapula down and toward the spine. First, you will need to put the scapula in such a position that the medial aspect of the scapula is exposed. It is a

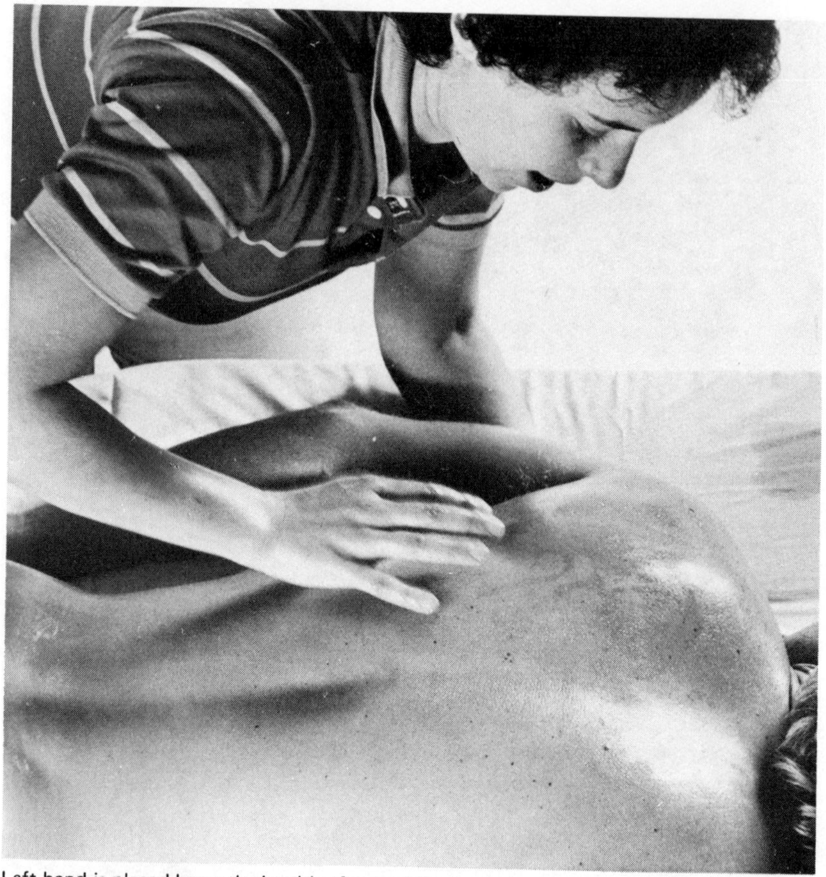

Left hand is placed beneath shoulder for working trapezius.

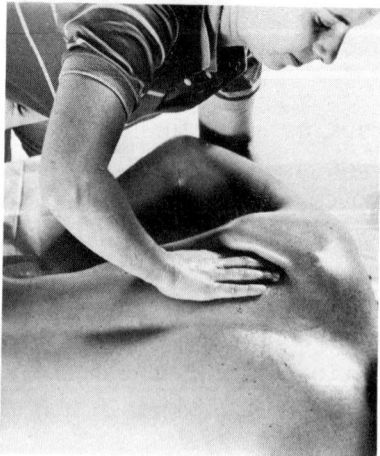

Fingers can trace the border of the
trapezius.

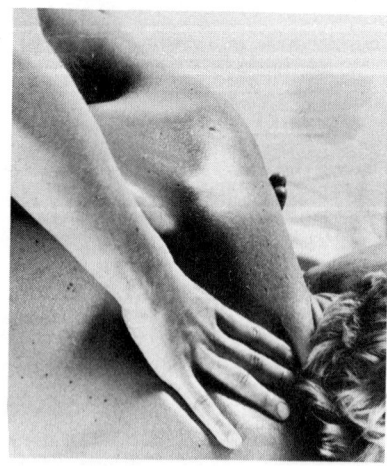

Your thumb can also be used.

triangular bone and the medial border is the one side facing and parallel to the spine.

To put the scapula in the best possible position, lift your partner's arm by the wrist, bending and supporting at the elbow, and bring it up across his low back so that his wrist is palm up on the spine. Stand at your partner's side or over his shoulder, supporting the elbow. Now reach your free hand under the shoulder, allowing his elbow to drop down to the table. You don't want to allow the humerus, the upper arm bone, to rotate or drop down excessively or to a point of discomfort; this is especially true for those who have had a dislocated shoulder. The scapula is exposed now. You can use your thumbs or the palm of your free

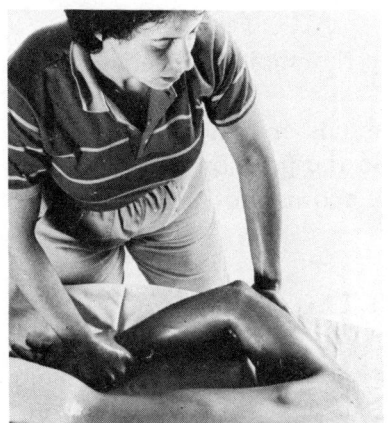

Move the arm to reposition the scapula for deep massage of rhomboid muscles.

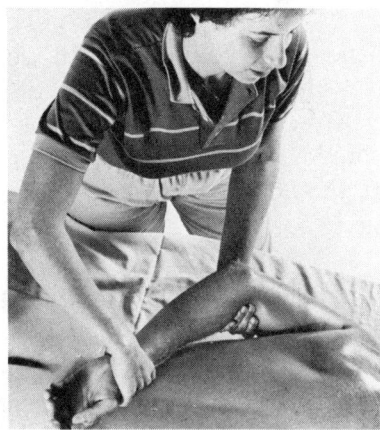

Place it behind your partner's back.

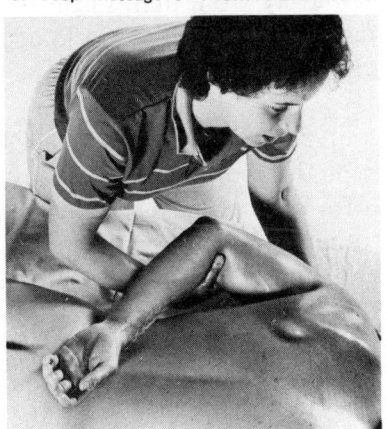

Position left hand under shoulder for support.

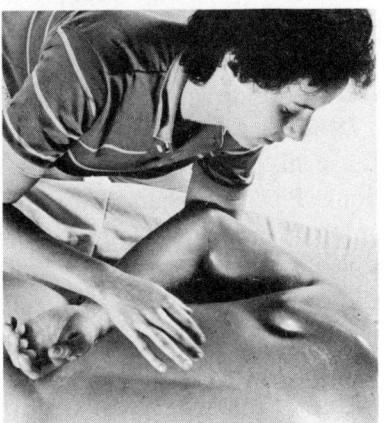

Medial of scapula is now exposed.

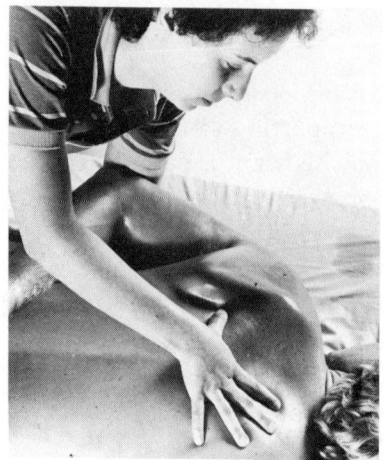
Use your thumb for deep pressure.

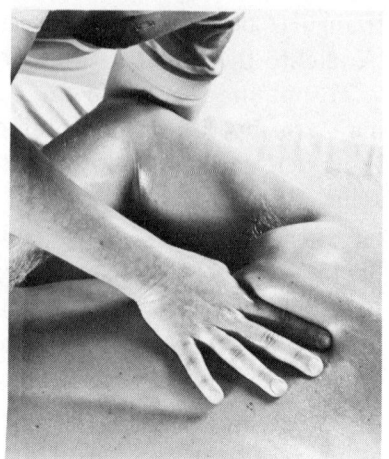
The fingers are also ideal for applying pressure.

hand—even your elbow—to work the rhomboid muscle and trapezius in the scapula notch.

After you've massaged the rhomboids and the trapezius, you should see a noticeable difference in the position of the scapula. It should protrude less on the back and might display some redness.

BACK OF THE LEGS

The hamstrings and calf muscles are easy to reach with your partner on his stomach. Concentrate in this area if you are working on an athlete whose sport calls for endurance leg strength.

Stand at your partner's side, facing away from him. Begin by stroking the lower back using effleurage, moving to the hip joints and then down the leg nearest you. Place the hands in the v-shape, and stroke down to the feet.

Now is a good time to stretch your partner's lower back, because his muscles will be relaxed from the work you've already done. Place one hand over the arch of a foot while anchoring the anterior part of the ankle with the other hand. Now pull the leg toward you using your body weight, making sure you support the ankle; do not yank on the leg.

Follow by doing the v-stroke, moving toward the heart to stimulate venous flow. First, grasp the back of the ankle nearest you with both hands. Now begin the v-stroke up the calf, over the

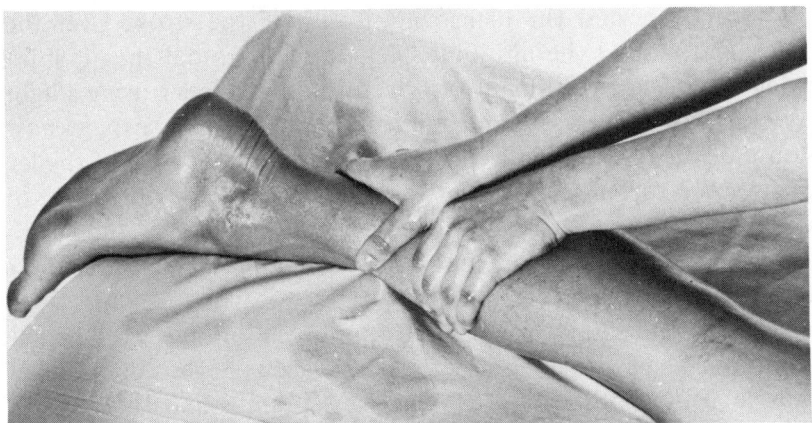

Stroke down leg with hands in v-shape.

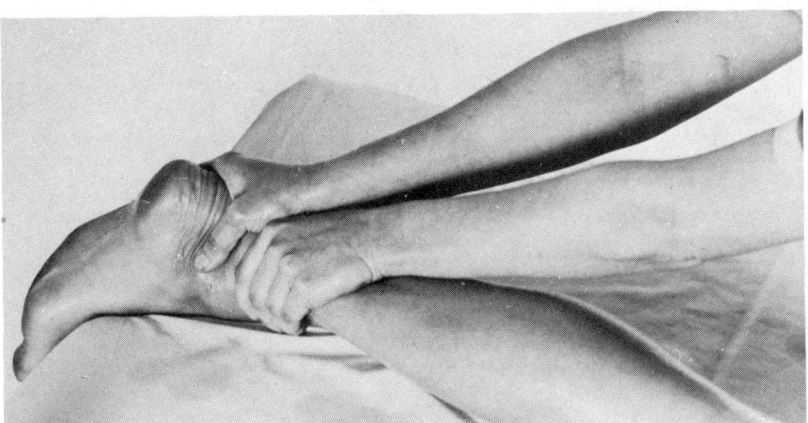

Finish stroke at the foot.

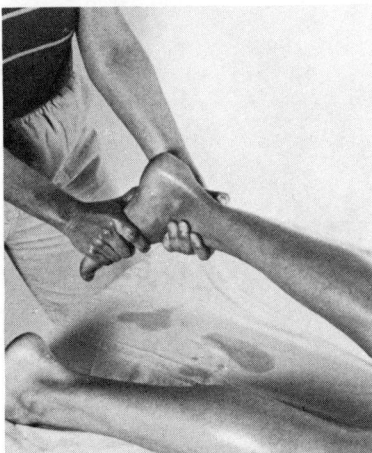

Pulling the foot will help stretch back muscles.

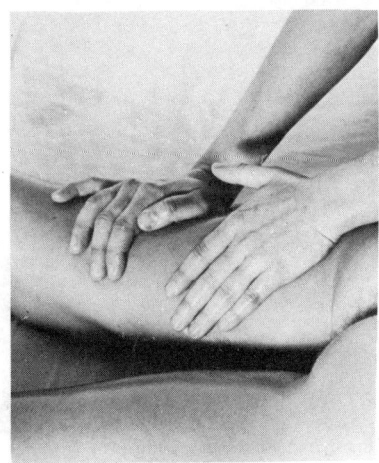

Hamstrings and calf muscles like deep pressure.

posterior knee and the hamstring. Continue the stroke over the pelvis and around the hip joint. Make circles around the hip joint using the heel of your hand. Now return down the leg using a light effleurage stroke, just enough pressure to let your partner know you are still touching him. You can return via the sides of the leg or over the top of the back of the leg. Move to the other side of the table now and massage the other leg. (Another method is to stroke both legs simultaneously while standing at your partner's feet.)

The circle-eight stroke can be employed on the calf, or the hand-over-hand stroke. Using the circle-eight stroke, lift the calf muscle using both hands. Spread your thumbs and fingers over the medial aspect of the calf, lifting as you knead.

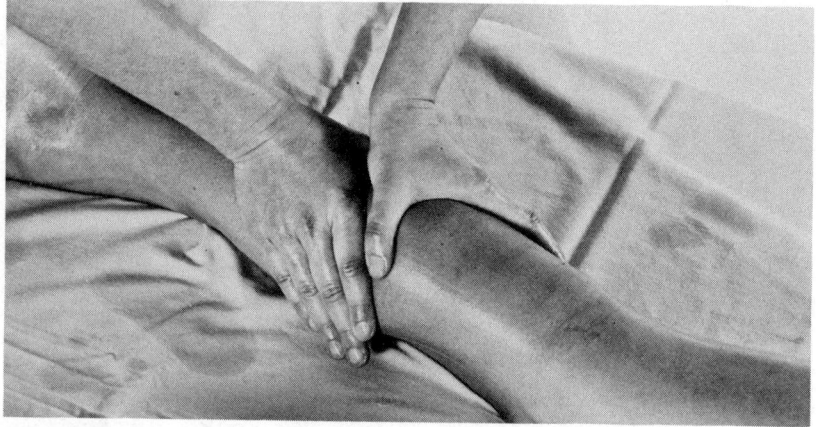

Return with the v-stroke.

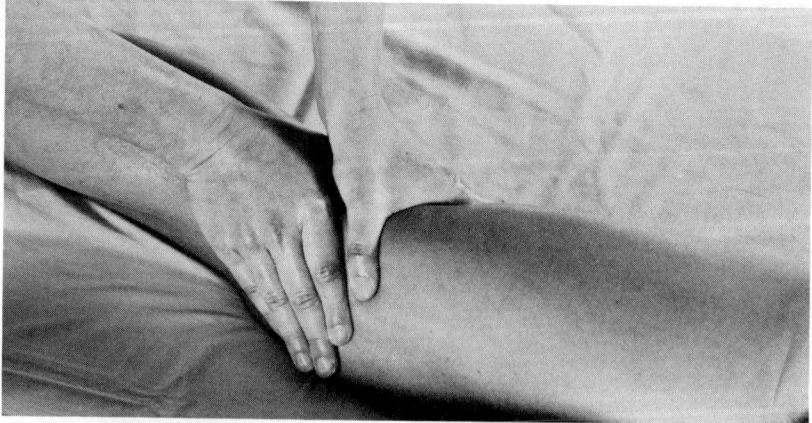

This stroke assists venous flow.

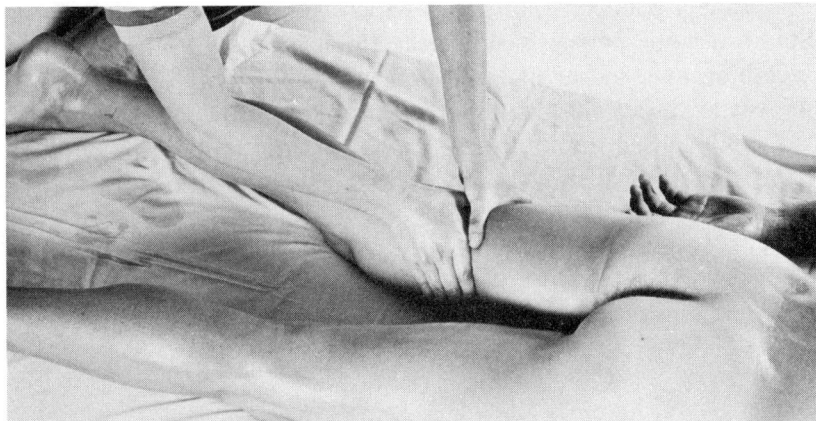

Your hands may separate on the wide part of hamstring.

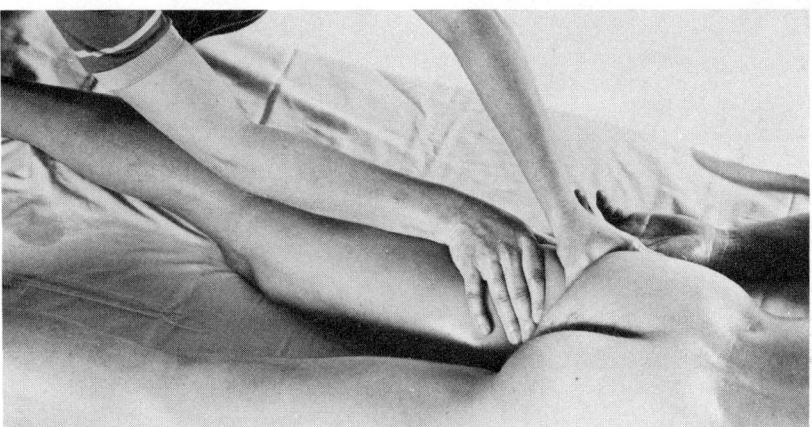

Use pressure on the posterior.

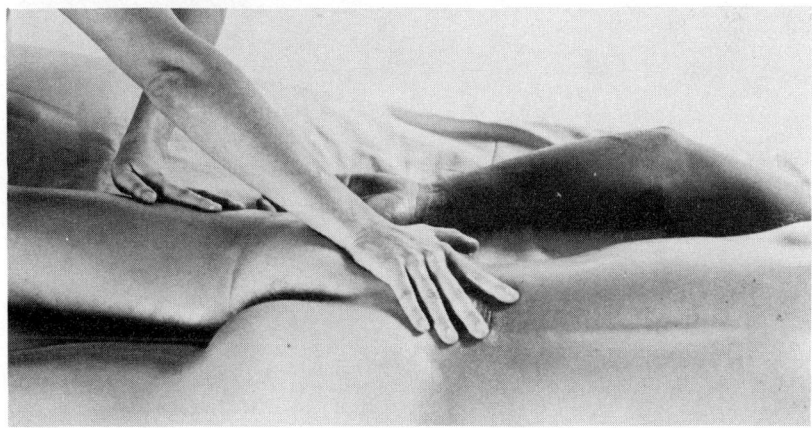

Use the heel of your hand and make circles.

Here is a good position from which to massage the calf muscle. Stand at your partner's side near the leg you're working on and face him, or stand at his feet. Grasp the ankle with one hand, lifting the lower leg and bending the knee. Support the lower leg with the ankle raised about twelve inches off the table. This puts the hamstring and calf muscles in their shortened, relaxed state. Now knead the calf with your free hand, using your fingertips, or stroke in small circles with your fingers and the palm of your hand. You can also work the hamstring.

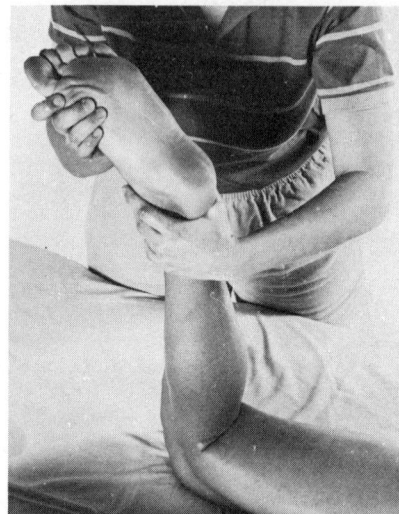

Lift the leg by the ankle to massage the calf. Knead the calf with your free hand.

Calf muscles are in their relaxed position here.

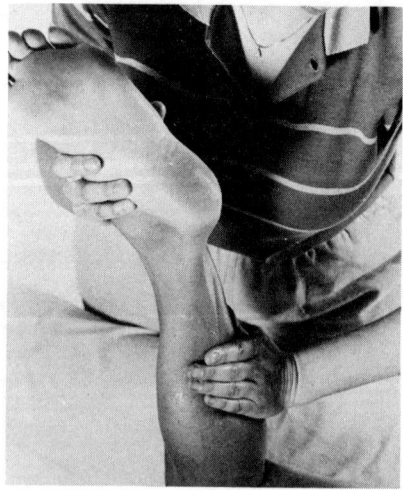

Occasionally, sitting on the massage table is the best position from which to work a body part or do a particular type of stroke, as with the harp stroke on the leg. Sit on the edge of the table facing your partner, one leg bent at the knee and resting on the table, the other leg straight, foot flat on the floor. You can rest your partner's right foot on your right shoulder by bending his knee and work this leg, while giving yourself a rest. Now use the heels of both of your hands to work the leg, much as you would pluck the strings of a harp. Work down the leg.

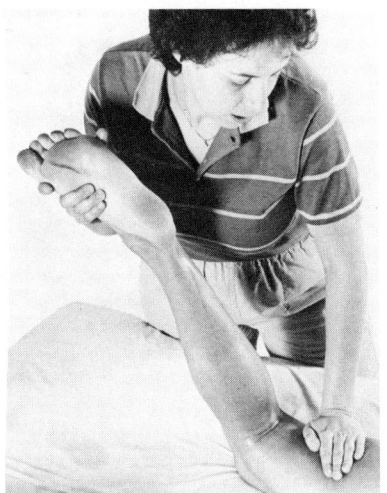
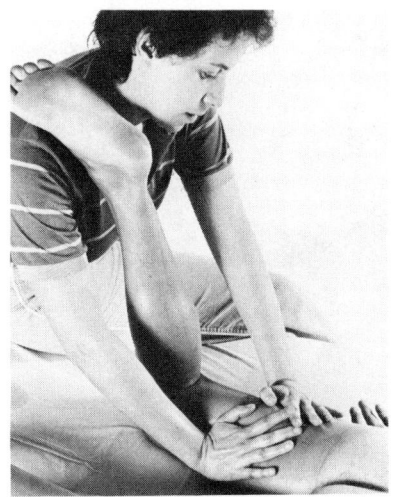

Move to the hamstrings. Use deep pressure. You may sit on the massage table to work the calf in this position. Your back gets a rest; you can also reach hamstrings.

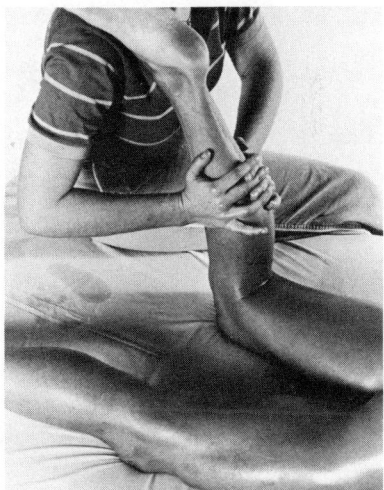

Now that you've loosened some of the leg muscles you can rotate the hip joint. Stand at your partner's side. With one hand grasp your partner's ankle nearest you. Place the other hand over the hip joint so you can feel the motion in the joint. Now lift the lower leg, knee bent, so that you can rotate the leg in circles. This motion is actually that of the hip rotating. Your finger and thumb should be able to pick up the head of the femur bone turning in the ball-and-socket joint as you slowly rotate the hip. Rotate the hip clockwise and then counterclockwise.

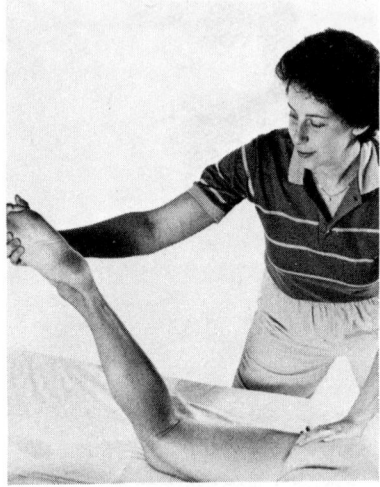

Stand next to your partner for the hip joint rotation.

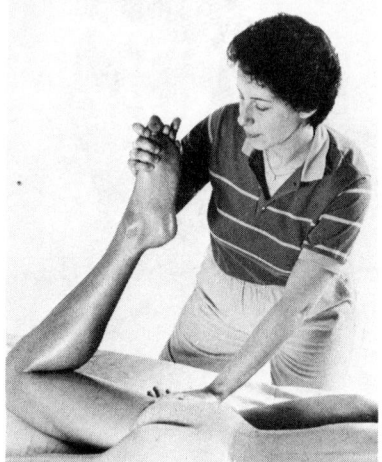

Hold the foot with one hand and move the leg in circles.

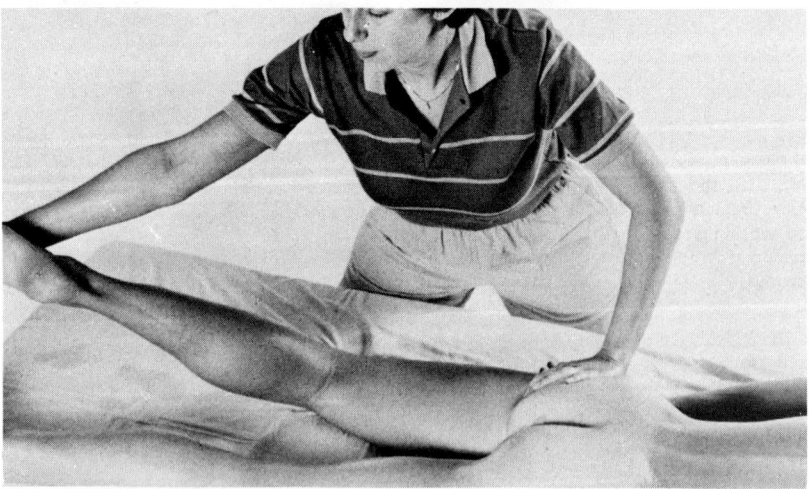

Your other hand should be placed over the hip joint.

Next try a quadriceps stretch on the leg you've been working. It is important that you keep the leg in a neutral position, in line with the rest of the body. Lift the left foot with your right hand, grasping the top of the ankle, and put your left hand on the fold of the knee, palm down. Bring the heel of the foot down toward the buttocks, holding the ankle with your right hand. Laying a hand in the fold of the knee guards against overstretching and isolates the stretch in the muscle, not in the knee joint. The paraspinal muscles of those who complain of tight backs may tighten noticeably during this stretch. If your partner has tight muscles you might not be able to stretch the leg sufficiently so that the heels of the feet touch the buttocks at the point of maximum stretch. To prevent the back muscles from tightening during this stretch, put your left hand on your partner's lower back, fingers

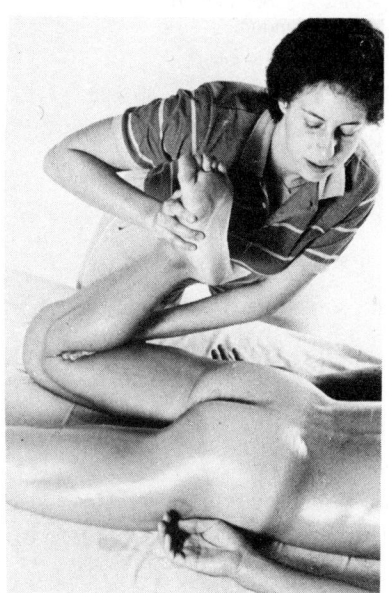

Now for a quadriceps stretch.

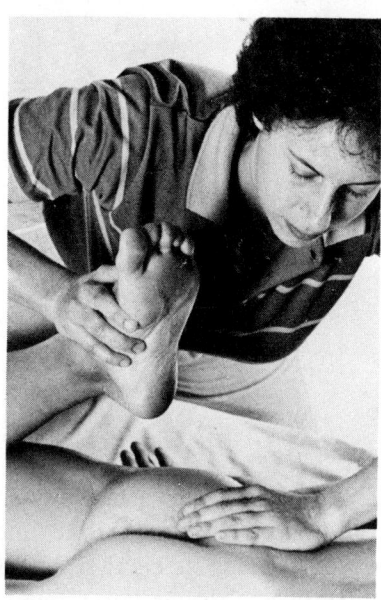

Without placing hand in the back of the knee, you can stretch the muscles farther.

pointing toward the feet. Your left hand was in the fold of the knee, so be extra cautious while stretching the leg. Hold the stretch for about fifteen seconds. Repeat with the other leg.

A final stretch on the lower leg can be done on the Achilles tendon. Basketball players, runners and women who wear high

heels are often in need of having this done. Stand at your partner's feet. Bend the knee and cup the heel in your hand. Use your
forearm of this same arm to lean into and push down on the metatarsals of the foot. The stretch will be felt in the calf.

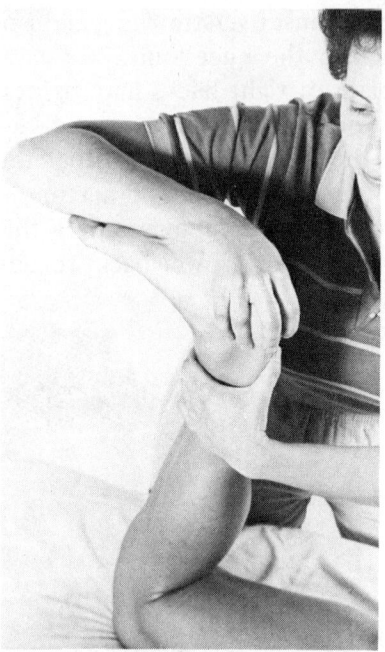

Here's a good method of stretching the
Achilles tendon.

HAMSTRINGS

The hamstrings are fleshy and thick and love deep pressure. Use
the hand-over-hand stroke, moving up toward the heart. Or, you
can use the circle-eight stroke.

Here is another good technique—a form of v-stroke. Stand at
your partner's side, facing him. Wrap both hands around the hamstring, where it attaches to the back of the knee. Your thumbs will
overlap, unless your partner has very large legs. Now push firmly
toward the posterior, following the contours of the hamstring
muscles. Hold your fingers loosely. The thumbs will probably
separate as you slowly move up the hamstring. Reverse the stroke
to return, using far less pressure.

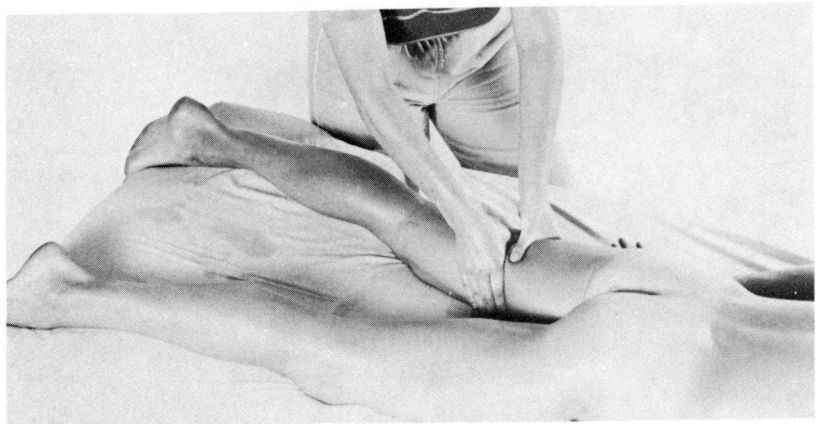

Use the v-stroke for the hamstrings.

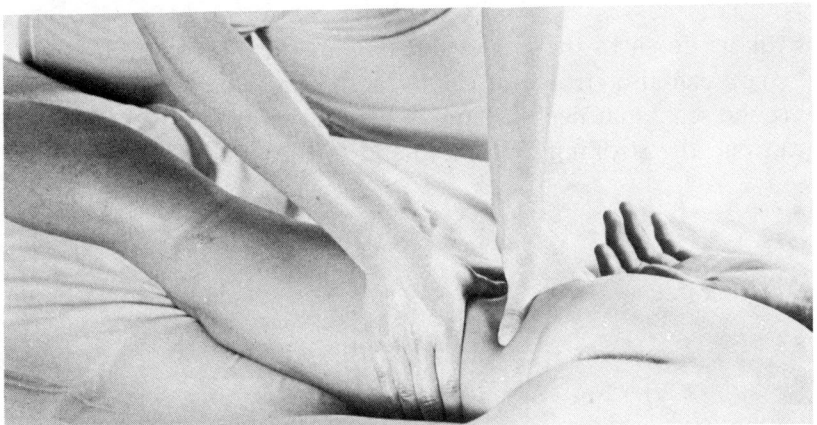

Hands should overlap.

The forearms are effective for massage of the hamstring. Re-main at your partner's side. The movement begins in the low-back area. Place both forearms here and bring them forearm-over-fore-arm over the hip and posterior. As your elbow reaches the side of the hip let your hands complete the stroke. Then return the fore-arms to the hamstring and repeat the movement.

We have finished with the massage of the back of your partner's body. Now we will finish with some strokes that unify the mas-sage. Finishing with the feet or the head is a common practice. In this situation you were last working on the legs, so finish with the feet. Stand at your partner's side. From here you can stroke the lower back using a light effleurage stroke. Bring in both legs,

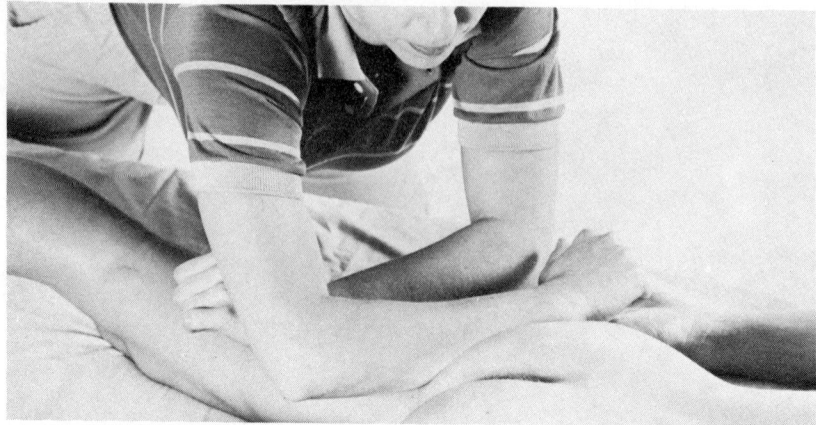

For deeper pressure, use your forearms on the hamstring.

stroking down to the ankles and holding them for several seconds.

You can also stroke up the back and finish on the head, kneading the scalp and neck. Standing behind your partner's head, you can end the stroking with one hand in the small of the back and

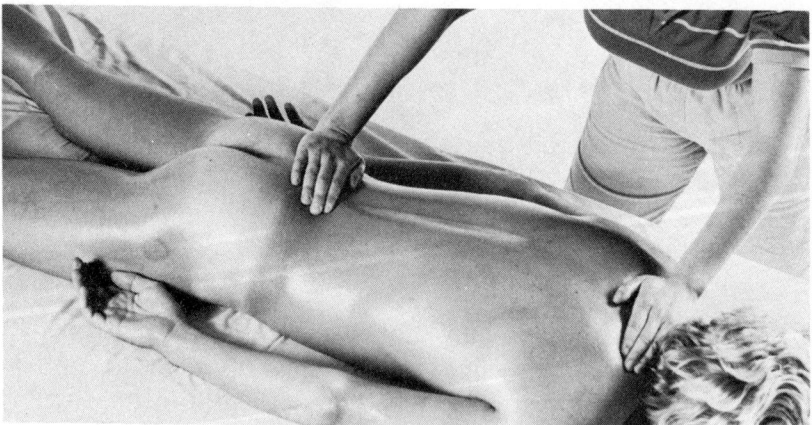

One position for finishing massage of the back — hands on lower back and neck.

one at the base of the neck. Or, you can stroke down the arms simultaneously, clasping your hands over your partner's hands and resting here for several seconds. The idea is to leave your partner with a feeling of total awareness, not for example, with thoughts directed at the big toe.

For people who tend to be flighty or "airy," try grounding them by finishing at the feet. People who are "heavy" or tend to have a mental burden might benefit by you finishing at the head, so that they will feel "lighter."

FRONT OF THE BODY

Have your partner turn over. There are dozens of ways to begin massage on the front of the body.

HEAD AND HAIR

Start at the head and work your way down the body. (You could also begin at the feet and work your way up, or any number of variations.) You should be standing behind your partner's head.

Massage the scalp by kneading it with your fingertips. Include the side of the head and the upper neck. You might try scratching your partner's head; mimic the action of drying wet hair with a towel.

Hair pulling can be very relaxing when done properly. Grasp a fistful of hair at its roots and then slide your hand gently through the hair. You can also hold the hair at its roots and pull back gently. Avoid pulling hair at the ends, because this can be painful. Now move your hands to the forehead.

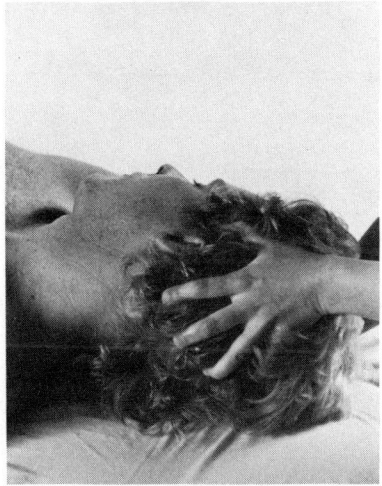

Massage the scalp using your fingertips.

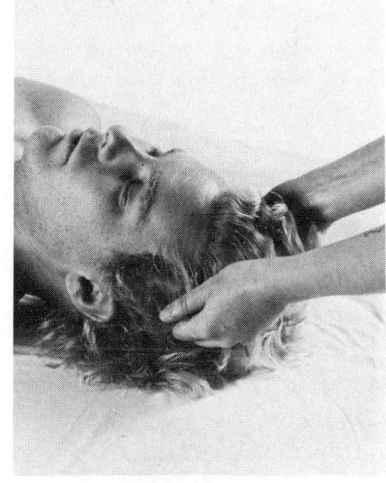

Hair pulling can be relaxing.

FACE

Begin at the forehead and work down or you may start at the chin and work up or start at the ears and work toward the nose. The possibilities for facial massage are endless.

Remember, contact lenses must be removed to massage over the eyes.

To start, interlock your fingers and rest them, palm down, on your partner's forehead. Now spread apart your arms, keeping them parallel with the floor. The heel of your hand, the palm and then fingers will stroke the forehead as you separate your

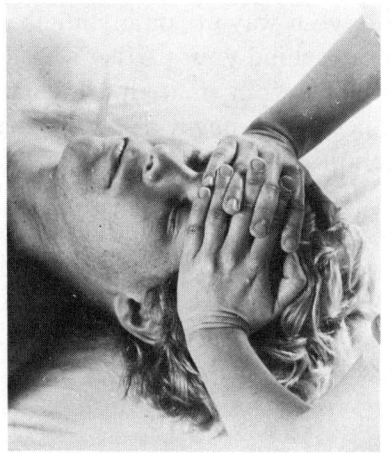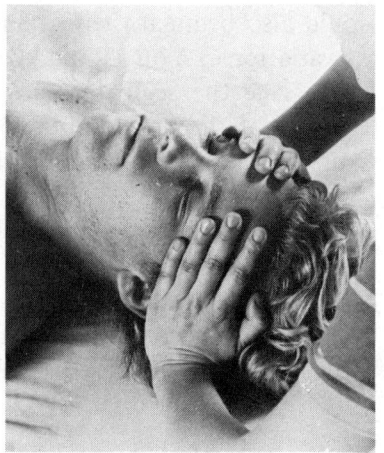

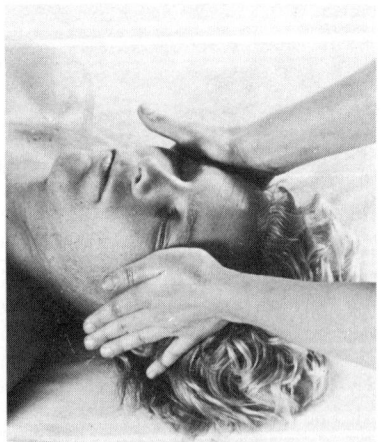

Begin stroke with fingers intertwined. Separate hands and move over the forehead. Bring your hands to the side of the head.

hands. You can do the same movement in reverse. Place the palms of your hands on your partner's head, just above the ears. Now bring your hands down simultaneously toward the forehead. The heel of your hand, the palm and finally the fingers will stroke the forehead. Next, the nose.

Place your thumbs on your partner's cheeks. Stroke up and across the bridge of the nose, keeping your thumbs parallel to one another. Move onto the forehead, thumbs touching. Now pull them apart, stroking over the forehead and finishing on the side of the head.

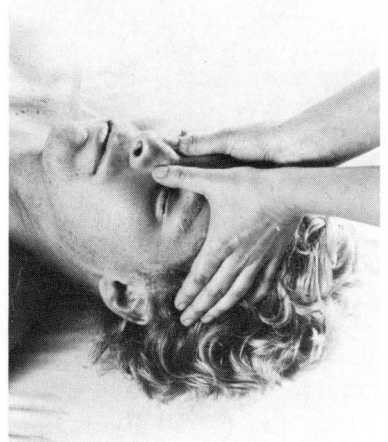
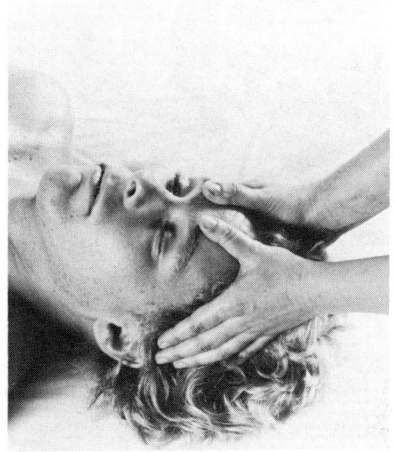

Place your thumbs over the bridge of your partner's nose. Spread your hands apart. Cover the entire forehead as you stroke.

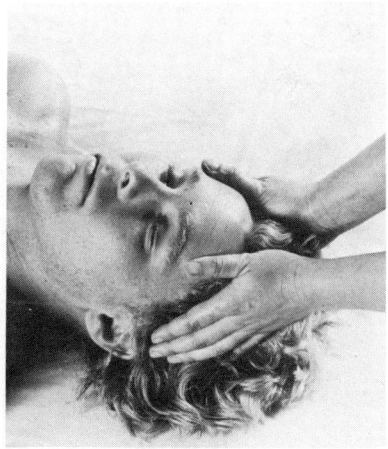

Now start the next stroke with your thumbs touching and resting on the bridge of the nose. Spread your thumbs over the eyebrows, ending the stroke at the temples. Now make small circles over the temples, using your thumbs.

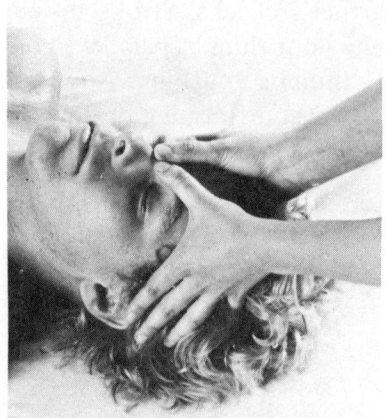

To stroke eyebrows, begin with thumbs on the bridge of the nose.

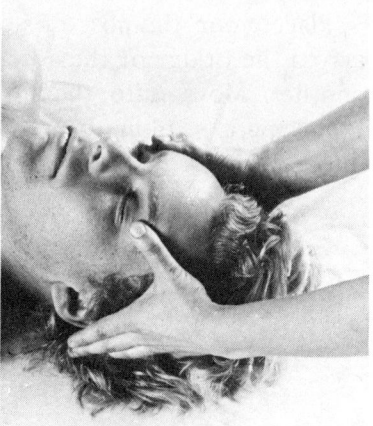

Spread your thumbs apart over the eyebrows.

While this is not a lesson in acupressure, there are several readily available points you can key on at the face. An acupressure point that releases tension and relieves minor headaches and stuffy sinuses is found just below the sixth chakra (Third Eye). Hold the fleshy part of your thumbs on this point for about six seconds.

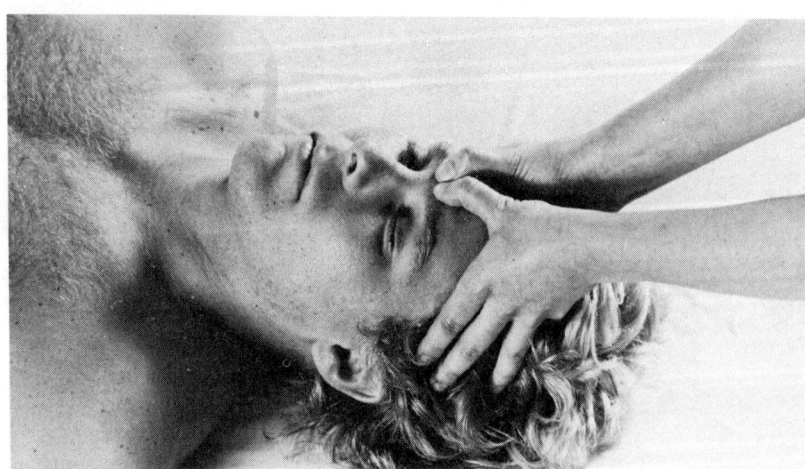

An acupressure point is above and between the eyes.

Or, place your index fingers over the eyebrows with your thumbs together and on the Third Eye.

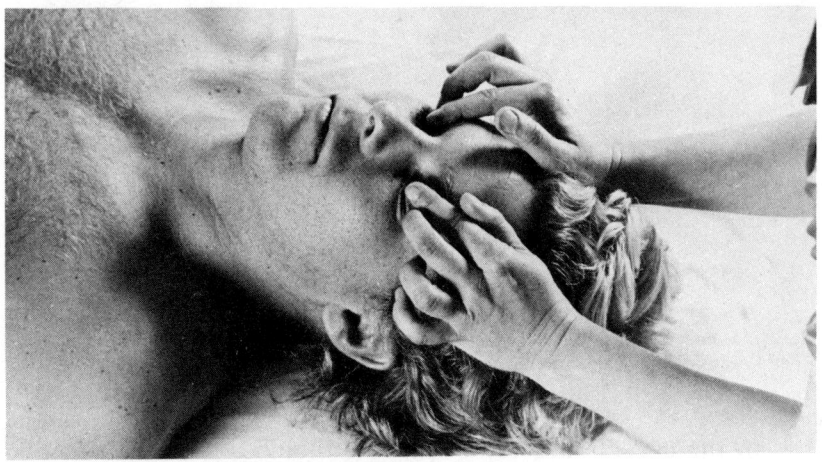

Anchor your hands and stroke the eyelids.

Stroking the eyelids with light effleurage can be quite soothing, but remember that the skin here is delicate and thin and that it is the only protection between your finger and your partner's eye. If your partner expresses dissatisfaction, discontinue massage here.

Try this movement for massaging the eyes. Place your fingers behind your partner's ears. Now place your thumbs over the eyes; starting from the bridge of the nose, glide them over the eye

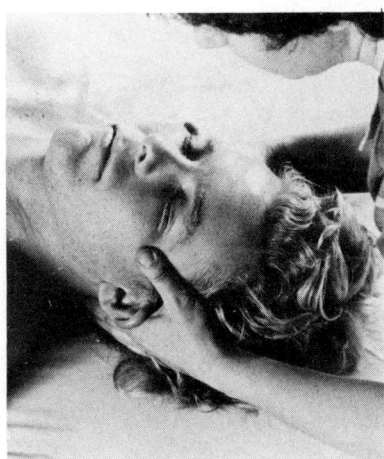

Now stroke down the side of the face.

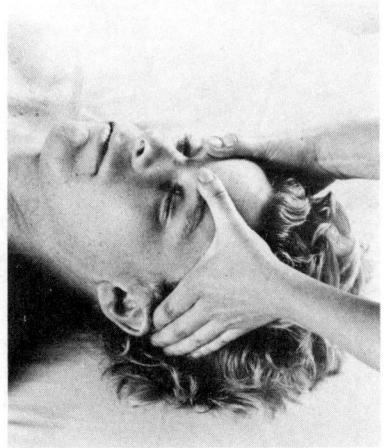

Trace the eyebrows once again.

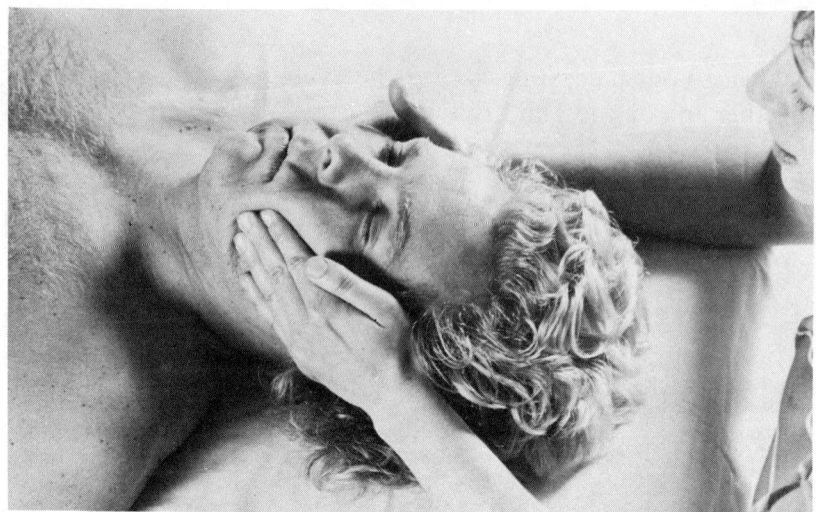

Then knead the masseter muscles with your fingers.

lids to the cheekbones. Now bring the thumbs down to the cheek-bones and make circles. Then trace the length of the cheekbones and move onto the jaw. Knead the masseter muscle, which extends from the jaw up to the cheekbone. This muscle is used for chewing and talking.

To massage your partner's chin, put your thumbs together in the middle of it. Place your fingers beneath the chin for support. Pull your thumbs apart, stroking to the hinge of the jaw. Now put the fingertips of your index fingers together over the top of the

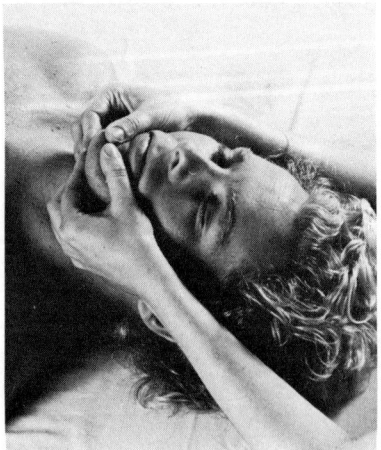

You can massage your partner's chin.

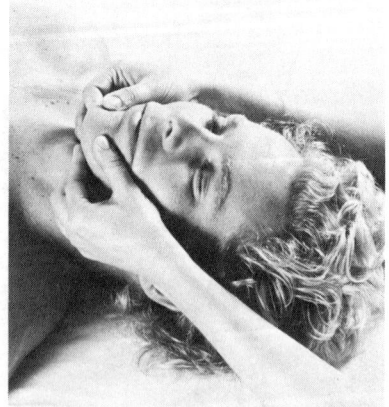

Place your thumbs together, then spread them apart.

lips, beneath the nostrils, and then pull them apart, crossing the edge of the cheeks.

To massage the throat use very light strokes, fingers spread and loose. Stroke up to the face.

Wrinkles on the face are caused by aging skin and weak facial muscles. Massage can help to tone the facial muscles and thus reduce wrinkling. Massage cannot rid you of wrinkles like some magic potient, but it will help condition the skin. Remember that most wrinkles run perpendicular to the muscles that control that area. If you are a constant worrier, there might be wrinkles running across your forehead. The frontalis muscle extends down the forehead, so you should massage it upward from the eyebrows. About the best advice for fighting wrinkles, besides having massage, is to avoid constant exposure to the sun, which causes a "pruning effect."

EARS

You will use your fingertips for most of the strokes. Trace the outlines of the ear and between the ridges and folds of skin, pulling gently. You won't need oil here. Avoid putting your fingers directly into the ear canal.

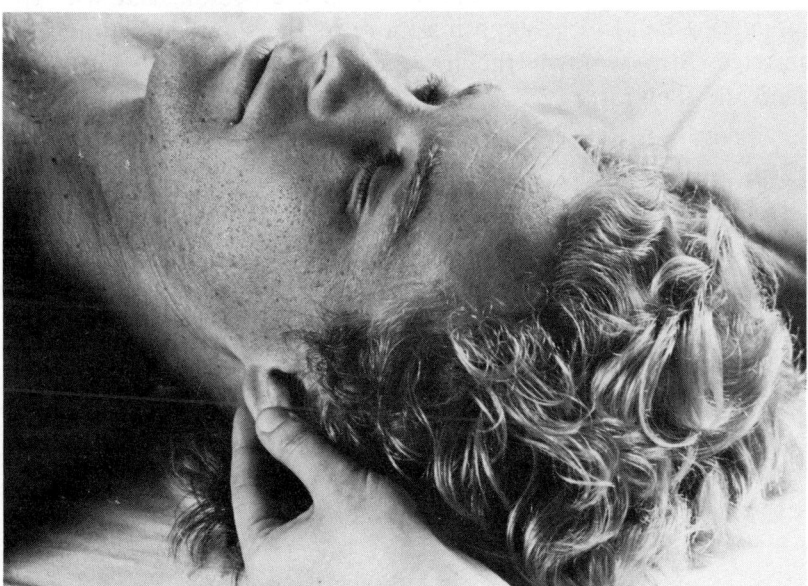

Trace the outlines of the ears with your fingertips.

NECK

Tension is a big part of modernday living and the neck is a highly receptive part of the body to these stresses and strains, in the form of tight muscles and neck spasms. A stiff neck will negatively influence your entire body's performance, even your thoughts. Massage strokes on the neck, no matter how basic, are effective in reducing this tension.

To begin, place your hands on the base of the neck and to the sides. Point your fingers toward your partner's feet. Stand behind your partner's head. Stroke toward yourself along the length of the neck until the weight of your partner's head is resting in both your hands. Now remove one hand and put it on the lower neck, while holding the head with the other hand. Stroke from the lower neck back up to where your other hand holds the head. Now let the stroking hand assume the supporting position for the head while you return your other free hand to the lower neck on the other side. Repeat the process with this hand. Do this movement a half-dozen times or more. This stroke creates the sensation of elongation, and is relaxing. You may also massage the top of the trapezius muscle, along the ridge of the shoulder, by extending the stroke to this area.

From this position, you can turn the head to one side with the supporting hand, thus exposing more of the shoulder and neck to massage. Stroke down the trapezius with the heel of your free hand and then return using your fingers.

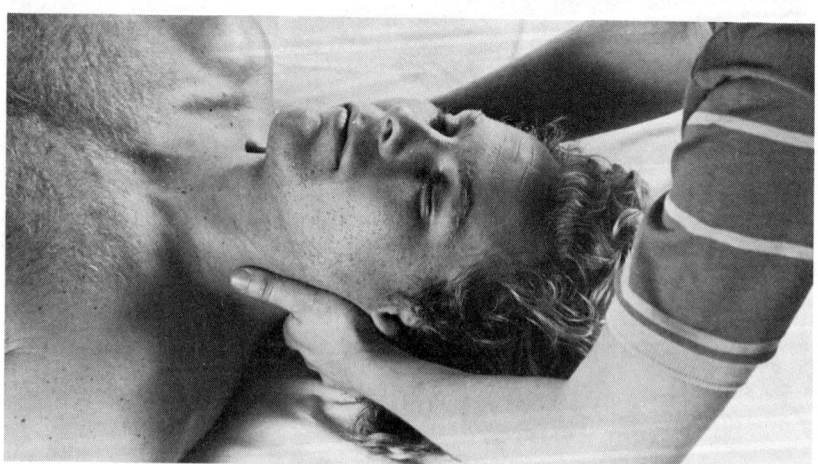

Place both hands beneath the neck.

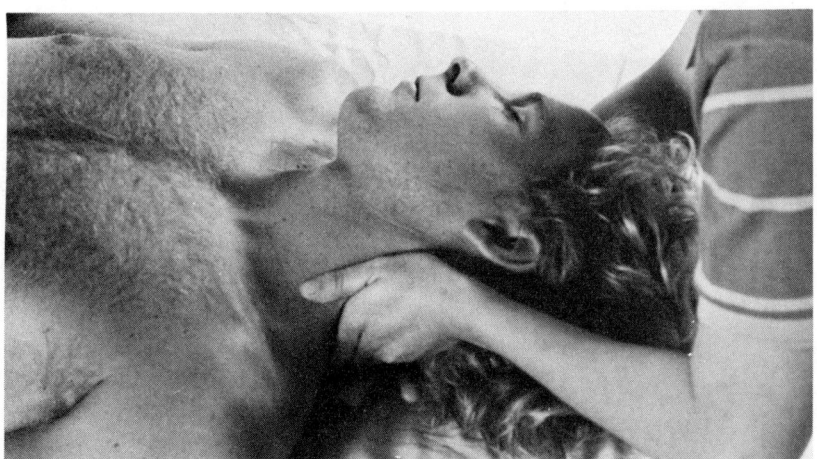

Switch hands as you work each side of the neck.

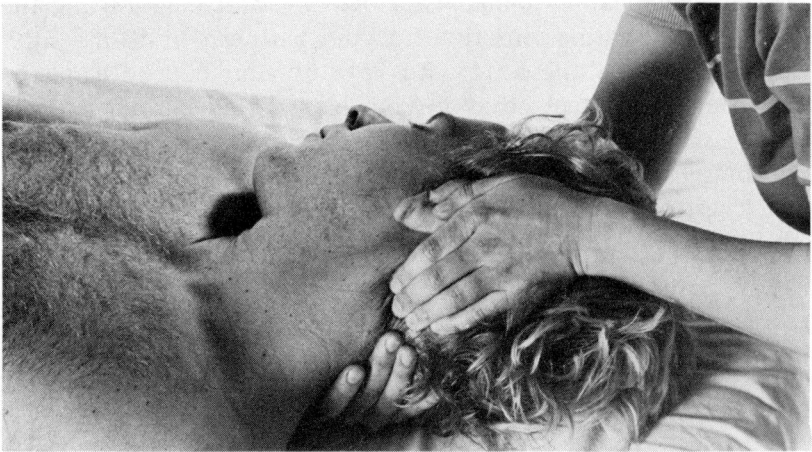

Use one hand to support the head, the other for stroking.

There are several acupressure points on the shoulders that will help relax the neck. One of them is located where the belly of the trapezius connects with the lower neck. Place the fleshy part of your thumbs on either side of the neck and press firmly into the muscle, anchoring your fingers on the clavicle. Your partner may experience a tingling sensation in the feet or hands. Get his reaction by asking him how he feels; you don't want to cause pain. Another acupressure point is on the neck a couple of inches up from the shoulder. Often these points are sore, so be sure you are tuned in to what your partner is feeling.

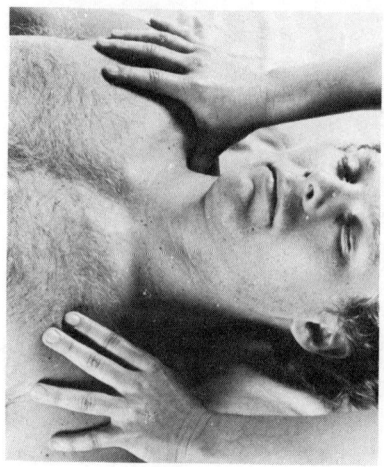

This is one acupressure point for the shoulders.

From acupressure points we move to stretching. Lifting the head up is a pleasing sensation for your partner, but lift it gently. Hold the back of the head with both of your cupped hands. If the head doesn't feel heavy in your hands, your partner is probably tensing his neck muscles, either consciously or unconsciously. Encourage him to let go and relax. You may lean the head on your chest or stomach, depending on how far forward your partner lies on the table. Place your hands, which are both free now, on the back of the shoulders and stroke up to the neck.

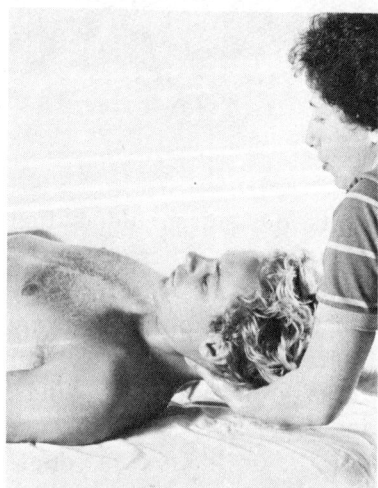

Lift the head off the table to stretch it.

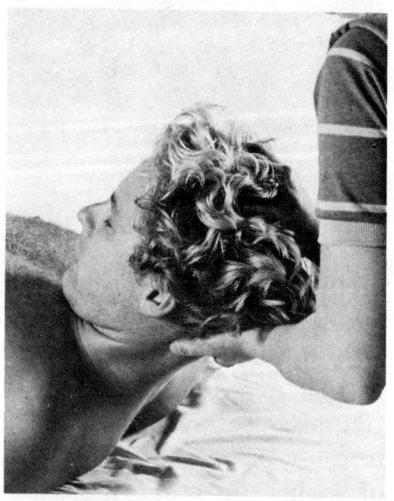

Pull on the head to stretch the neck muscles.

UPPER BODY

Remain standing in front of your partner's head for the following strokes. Place your hands on your partner's shoulders, fingers pointing toward his feet or navel and your thumbs pointing down against his back. Now apply pressure horizontally to the shoulder (toward the feet) but don't move the hands. Alternate pressure from one shoulder to the other; your partner's neck will probably rock back and forth.

The main stroke for the front torso begins with both hands on the clavicle. Stand in front of your partner. Move your hands lightly over the chest, fingers loosely together following the contours of the body. Once past the chest, fan your fingers over the ribs and down as far as you can reach. Bring your hands back up along the sides and to the armpits, pivoting at the shoulders and moving onto the neck. Finish at the occiput. This is one long, full body stroke.

There are variations. Place your hands together at the base of the throat. Bring both of them down to the chest. At the point of farthest extension, separate your hands and move them to your partner's sides. Make circles and return your hands up the body. Once in line with the chest, bring the hands back together and pull them between the breasts, separating again once past the breasts (for men, the same stroke applies). Finish at the shoulders. Now move your hands down your partner's arms and when you reach his hands, hold your hands over his for several seconds.

You can also start at the hips and pull your hands up the center of the body, then move them to the sides of the body, hands separating at the base of the shoulders and then finishing up on the back of the neck and head.

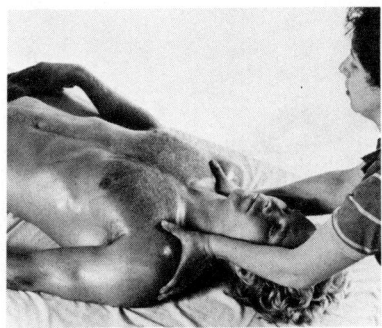

A stroke for the upper torso begins at the shoulders.

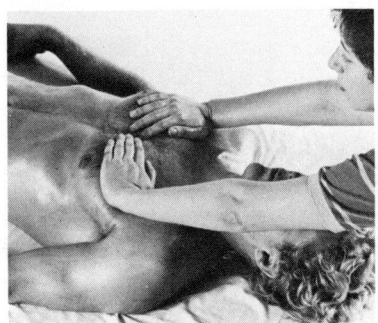

Separate your hands and move down the torso.

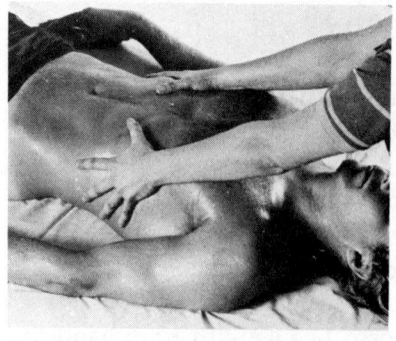

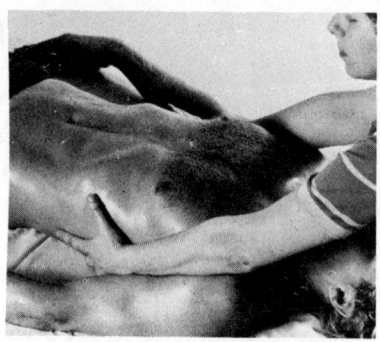

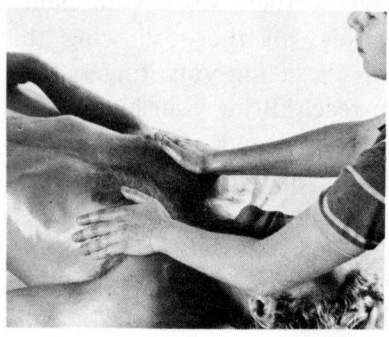

Stop before reaching the stomach and return with the hands spread on both sides of the body. Trace the edge of each armpit as you return. For the full torso stroke, begin at the shoulders. Spread your hands and move down to the hips. Stroke over the sides of the hips. Return with your hands on the sides of the body. Finish with your hands back on the chest.

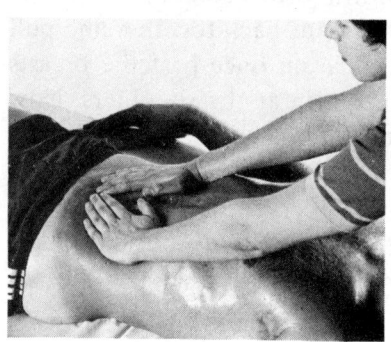

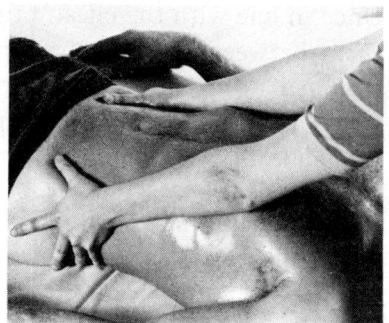

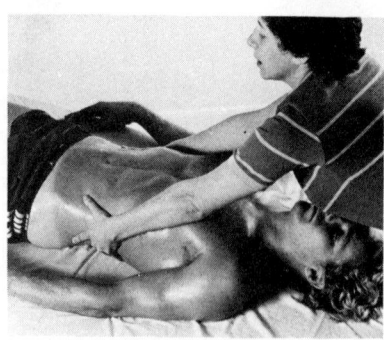

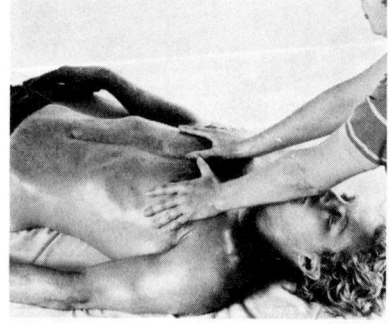

CHEST

Begin with the hand-over-hand stroke. Stand at your partner's side, reaching over to the opposite hip, facing away from him. Begin the movement at the hip and follow the contour of the ribs, pulling to the center of the chest and from there on up to the shoulders; include the armpit. Repeat this stroke several times. You can then move to the other side of the table and continue pulling with your hands on the opposite side or remain on the same side of the table and push up on this side of the body, moving from your partner's side to the center of the body.

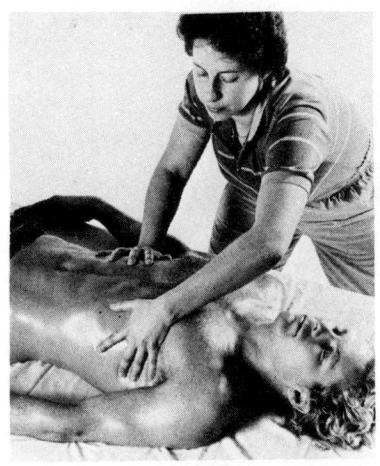

Stand at your partner's side for the hand-over-hand chest stroke. Bring each hand down to the side opposite you. Then pull up over the chest, alternating hands.

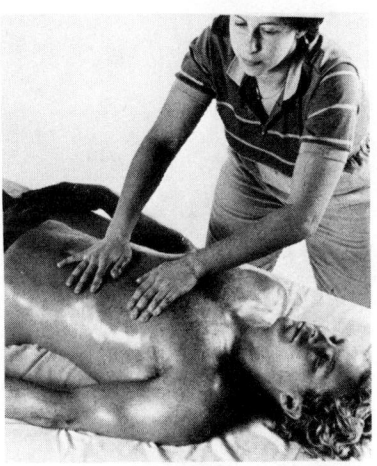

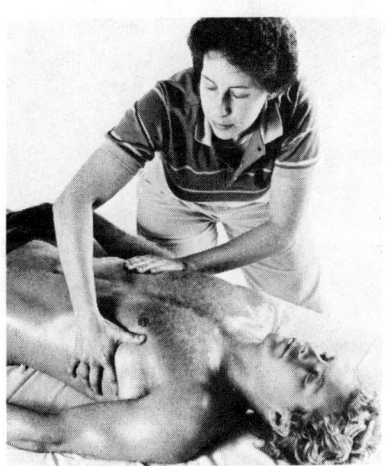

The diamond stroke begins on the chest and extends to the pelvis. Stand at your partner's side facing him. Place your thumbs on the sternum. Stroke just below the ribs with your thumbs; then extend your fingers down and beneath the lower back. Pull them up slightly now—you don't want to be lifting—and stroke to the pelvis, bringing your thumbs and fingers back to the top of the pelvis and over the pubic arch, and finally, return your hands to the sternum.

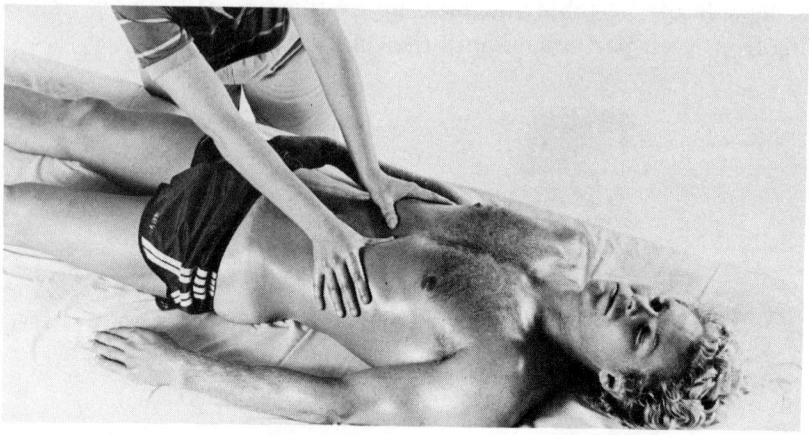

Start the diamond stroke with hands on the chest.

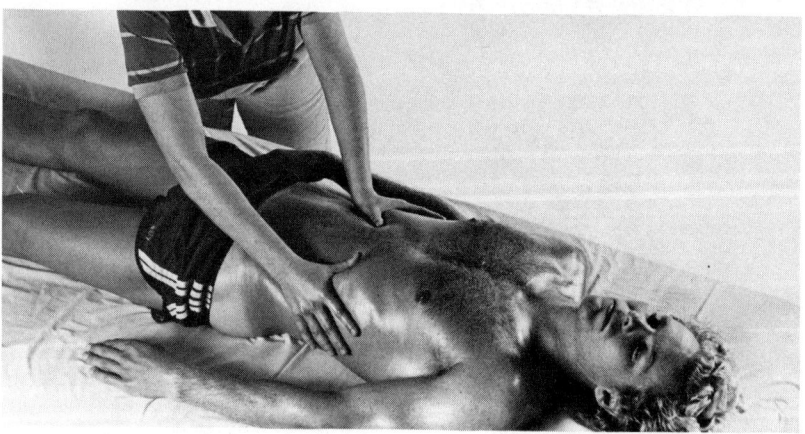

Separate your hands at the stomach.

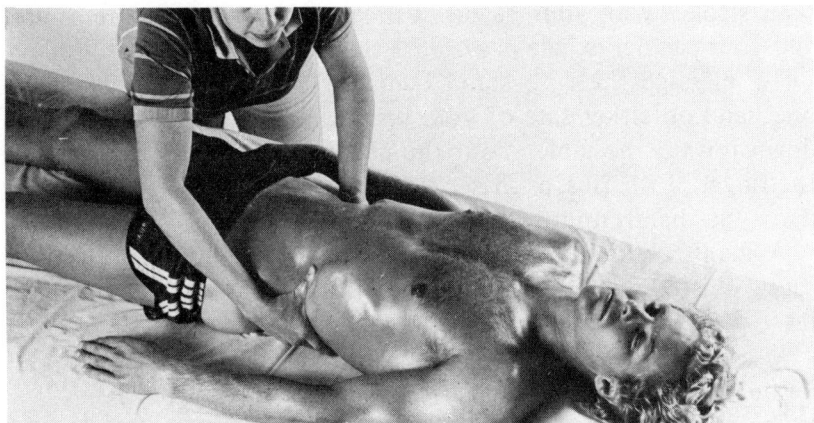

Place both hands underneath your partner's side and then pull gently.

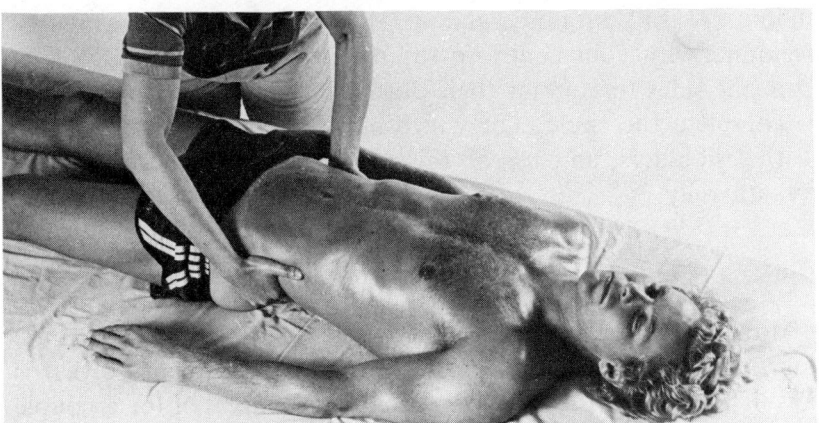

Move your hands around the pelvis. Don't lift up the back.

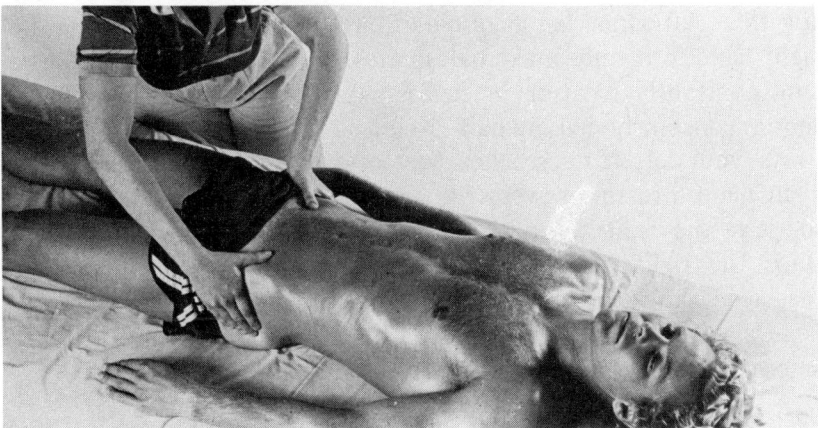

Return your hands to the sternum.

While working the upper chest and the ribs try to coordinate your strokes with your partner's breathing. Exert pressure as you and your partner exhale.

To massage the ribs, stand behind your partner's head. Place one hand on either side of your partner with your fingers pointed down toward the table. Your thumb or fingers can trace between the ridges of the ribs, as they extend to the sides of the body; then draw your hands up toward the sternum.

A man's chest can be treated like any large body surface, because it is composed primarily of muscle tissue, bone and some fat.

Massage of a woman's breast is a different matter, but should not be avoided. There are specific strokes for breasts.

The aim of breast massage is to counter the weight of gravity. Stand behind your partner's head. Always work with your hands pulling toward your body, and up. Make circles around the breasts, beginning with your hands on top of either breast and pulling up from the sides to counter their outward sag as you swing back up to complete the circle. You can bring your hands all the way up to the shoulders, and repeat this motion several times. Use light pressure only.

STOMACH

Move to your partner's side to work on the stomach. Rotate your hands clockwise around the colon's traverse, because that is how it is wound. Ideally your partner hasn't eaten for a couple hours preceding the massage.

Start with your left hand, palm down and fingers held loosely together. After making a couple of circles, begin incorporating the right hand, but only make half-circles. Pretend the left hand is the sun, constantly rotating in circles, while the right hand is a half-moon, constantly making half-circles.

As your left hand reaches the top of the stomach, bring the right hand into the movement, placing it on the left hip and moving it to the right hip, with your left hand following right behind. Once the right hand reaches the right hip, remove it, having massaged the lower half of the stomach. Continue with this procedure until you get the hang of it, i.e., when your motions are smooth. Now stroke back up to the shoulders.

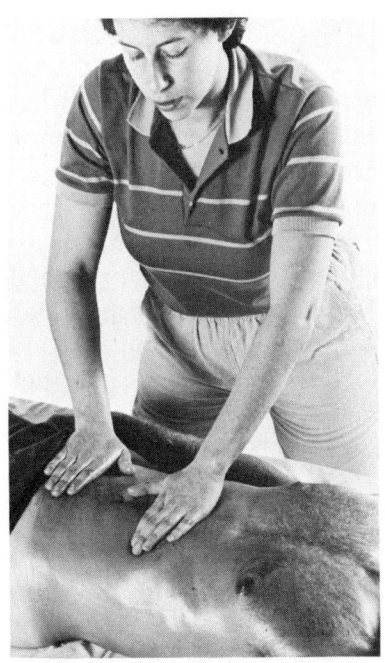

Place both hands together for the stomach massage.

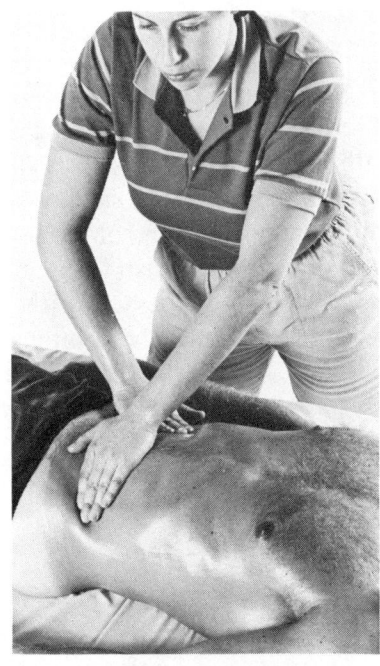

One hand will make full circles.

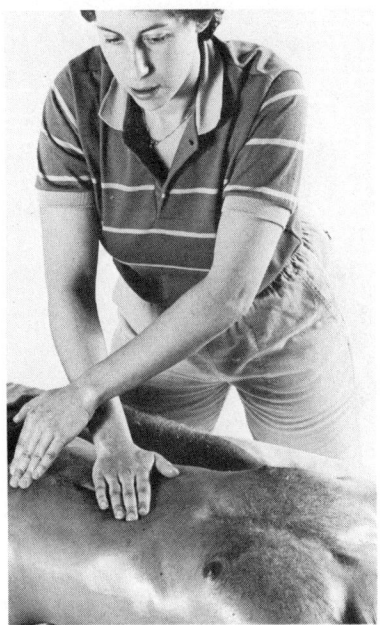

Make half-circles with the other hand.

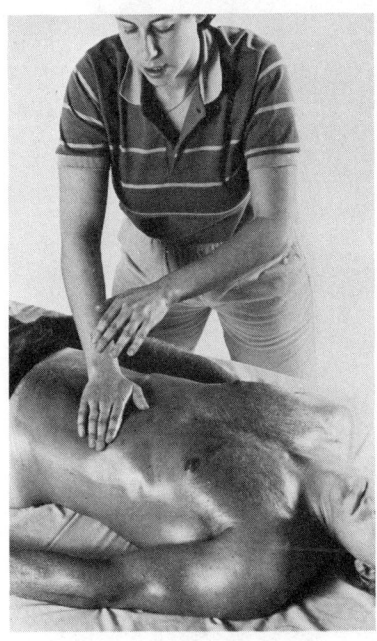

Learn to coordinate your movements here.

ARMS

Stand at your partner's side, facing him. Rest one hand on the edge of the shoulder, palm up and fingers extended. Place the other hand palm down on the top of the shoulder with fingers also extended. Now stroke from the shoulder to the hand, while enveloping the arm, finishing at the fingertips. To return, anchor the arm at the wrist with one hand and then stroke up to and over the top of the arm with your free hand in the v-shape. Glide your thumb into the armpit, pivoting around the shoulders and sliding back down the outside of the arm. Alternate hands, but this time glide your fingers into the armpit and return down the

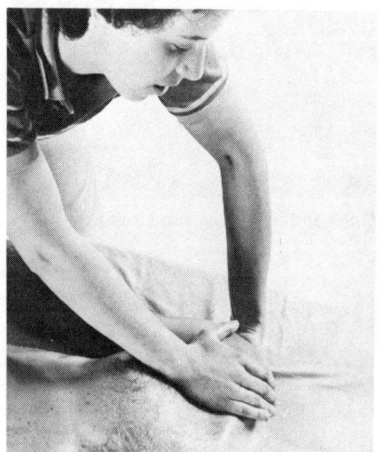

Start a full arm stroke at the shoulder.

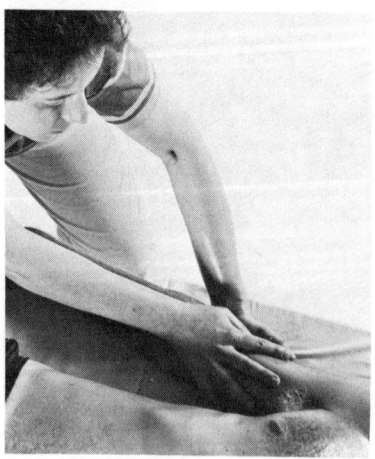

Bring both hands down the length of the arm.

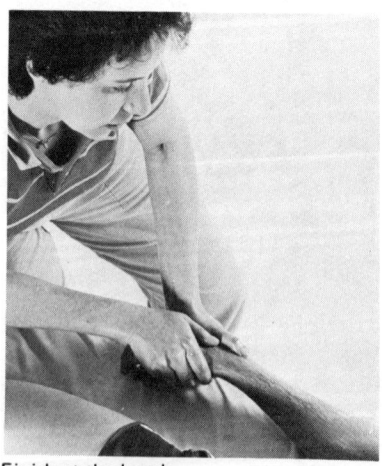

Finish at the hands.

inside of the arm.

You have been working the arms as they rest on the table, but now hold one arm in the air to conduct different movements and assist venous drainage. Lift the arm closest to you. The ability to extend the arm varies from person to person, but never pull to the point of causing pain to your partner. Rest your partner's left arm on your shoulder. Now your hands are free to knead the arm between the elbow and shoulder.

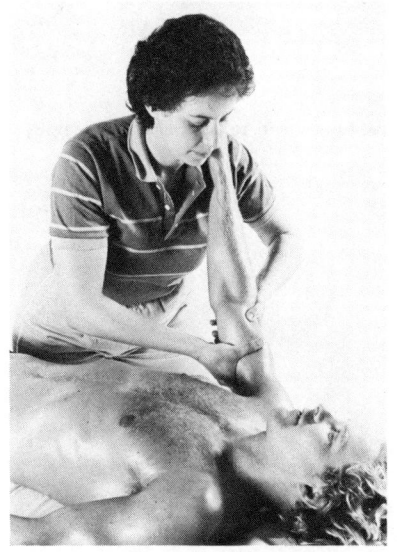

Hold the arm on your shoulder to work the biceps.

The next stretch is a good one for your partner's side, affecting the latissimus dorsi and intercostales. Hold the arm out and over your partner's head, at the wrist, elbow slightly flexed. Use your free hand to travel down the side of the body, starting at the arm. Move around the hips, pushing away at the hips toward the feet, circling around and then stretching all the way back up by pulling on the arm and pushing against the body using your stroking hand. Bend the arm at the elbow slightly more and stroke down the arm, around the breast and then back up over the armpit. Return your partner's arm to rest on your shoulder. Place one hand on the table, supporting your partner's shoulder. With your free hand, pull up on and knead the muscles between the elbow and hand. Or, you can use kneading, both hands rotating the shoulder.

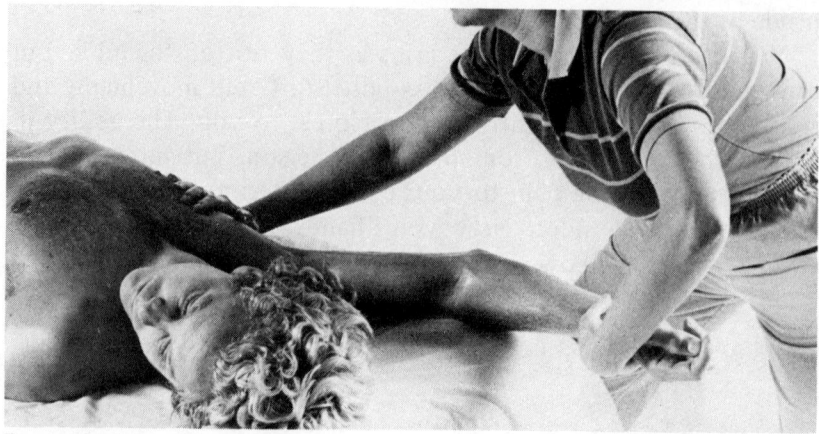

To stretch the arm, pull it back over the head. Use one hand to push against the body.

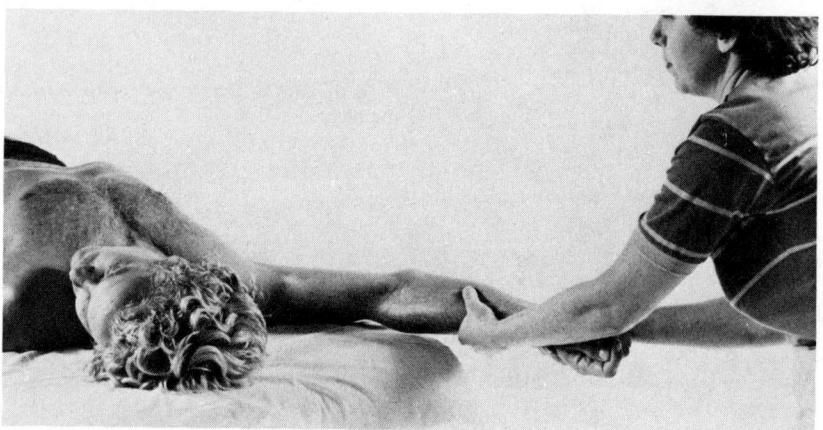

Now you can pull the arm with both hands.

Now try the harp stroke. Rest your partner's wrist against your stomach. Make a loose fist with your hands and massage down the forearm using your thumbs; alternate hands.

This is an easy arm stretch. Take your partner's arm by the wrist using both hands and pull it straight up in the air. Now free one hand and lightly stroke with it down to his shoulder. Then stroke back up using the free hand.

Here is a variation for shoulder work. Place the extended arm across your partner's chest. You can now reach under the shoulder of that arm with both hands. Palms are up and fingers are extended. Pull out your hands to stretch the back muscles.

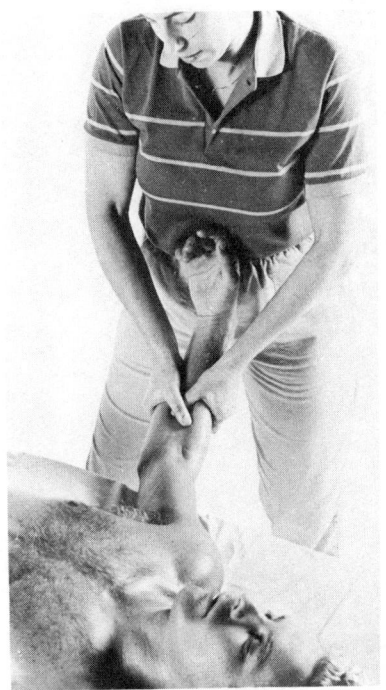

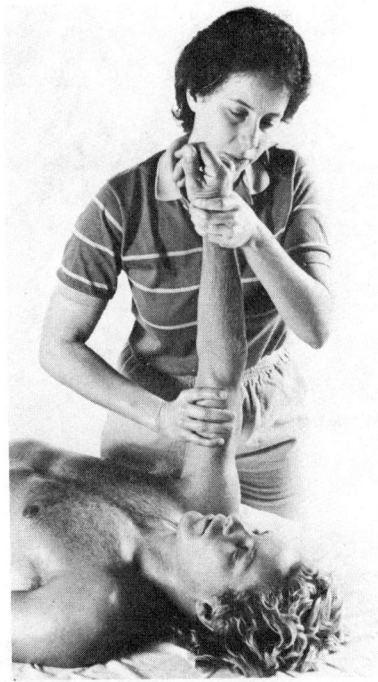

Use the harp stroke to work the lower arm.

Pull the arm up in the air with both hands to stretch it.

HANDS

The hands are ideal surfaces on which to create your own strokes and you can use considerable pressure on their fleshy side. Stand at your partner's side. Extend his arm over the side of the table and support it at the wrist with one hand. Place his thumb between the thumb and first finger of your free hand. Draw your finger and thumb away from your partner as you stroke the thumb. Repeat this stroke for all of the fingers, using a slight wringing or corkscrew action. Wiggle the joints as you stroke, always moving from the base to the tip of the finger.

Now work the back of the hand. Rest your partner's palm on your fingers, stroking using your thumbs. Notice the tiny bones and strands of ligaments and tendons. You can stroke between the ridges with your fingers or use circular motions with your thumb.

Now stretch the palm. Hold your partner's hand palm up with both of your hands. Wrap your fingers around the back of the

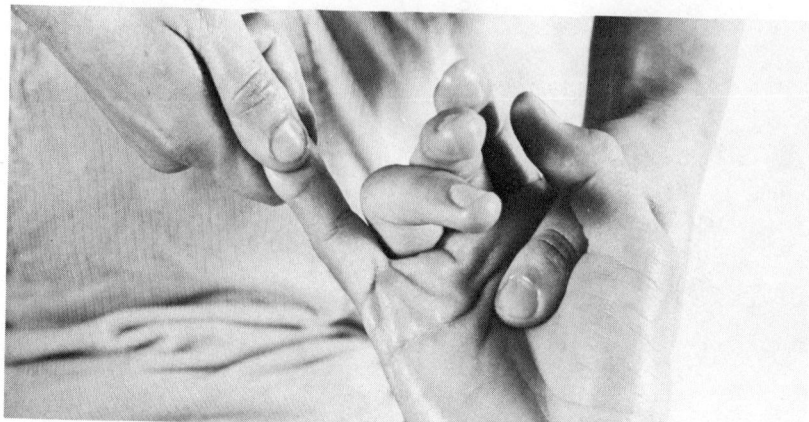

Work the fingers of the hands.

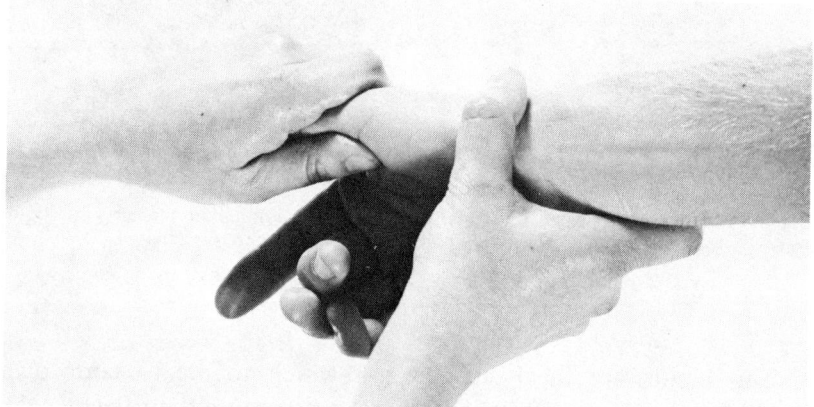

Use a slight twisting motion as you pull the fingers and thumbs.

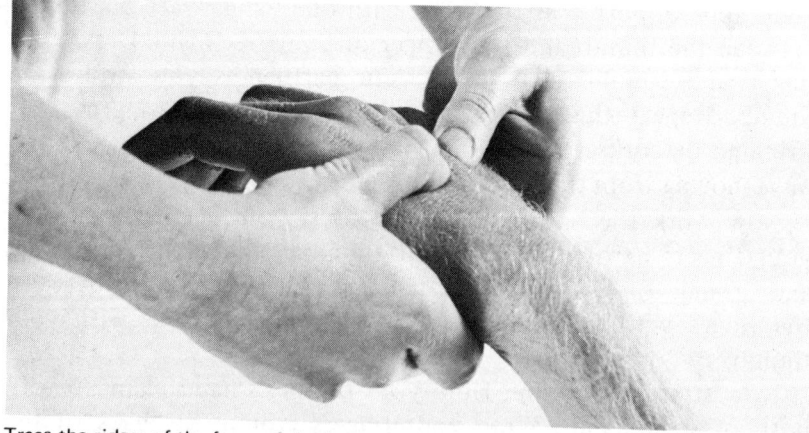

Trace the ridges of the front of the hand.

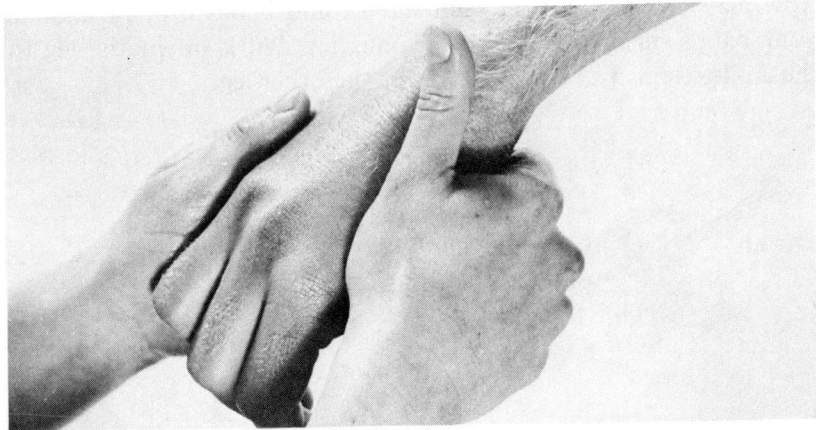

Use your thumbs to work the front of the hand.

hand and place the butt of your thumbs against his palm on both sides. Now press firmly against the palm, using the entire length of your thumbs, bracing the back of the hand with your fingers. Spread the palm by moving your thumbs apart.

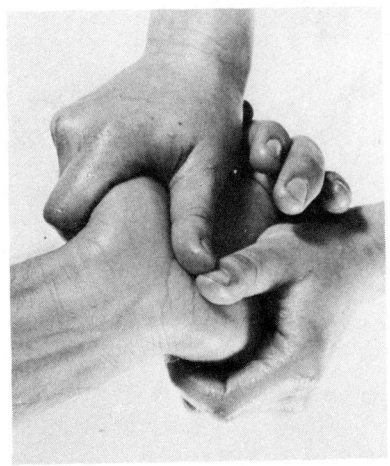

Place your thumbs together to spread the hand.

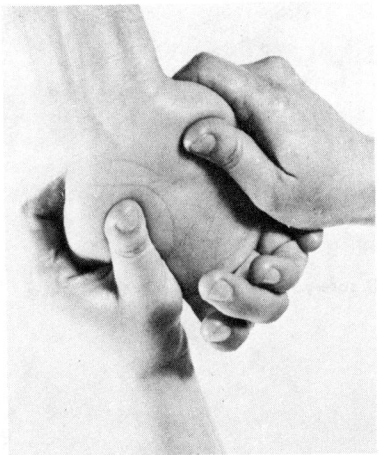

Stretch the hand as your thumbs separate.

FRONT OF LEGS

Move to your partner's side, facing him. Beginning from the hip, stroke down the leg using the hand-over-hand movement. Return with a light effleurage stroke and repeat several times.

Now place both hands on each side of and beneath one leg. Slide your hands out here, lifting the muscles. Work down the leg to the ankle. Repeat this procedure for the other leg.

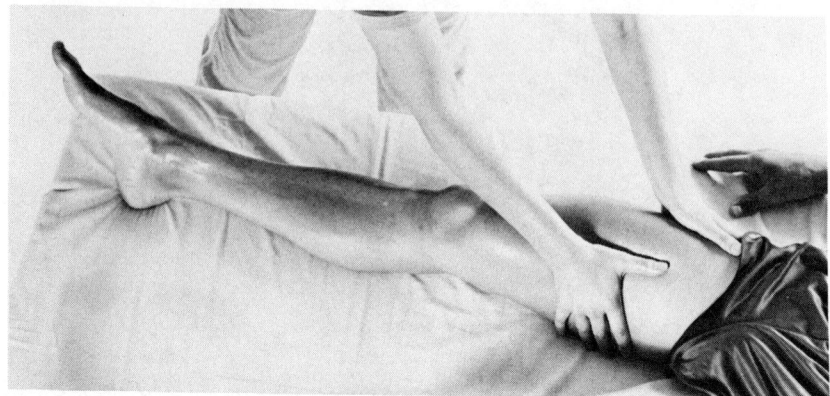

Use hand-over-hand effleurage to work the entire leg.

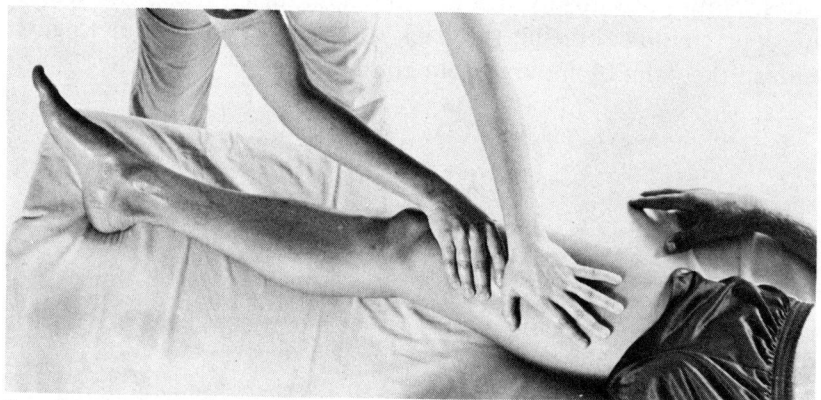

Be sure you use enough oil on hairy legs.

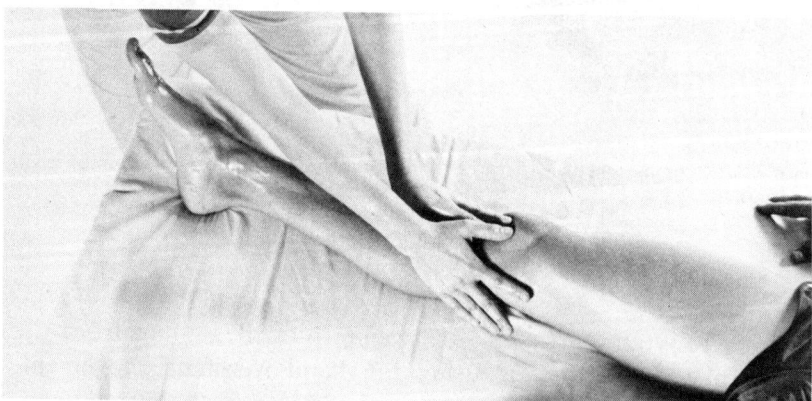

Stroke down the ankle.

You can use the heel of your hand, your thumbs, a v-shape and circle motions up and down the legs. If your partner has hairy legs be sure to use plenty of oil.

Now for some stretching. Hold one of your partner's ankles by one hand while standing behind his feet. Then pull, thus stretching the lower back. Be gentle. Do it to the other leg.

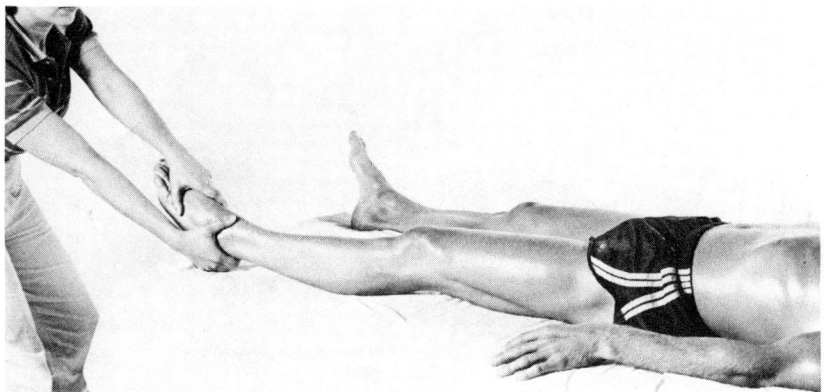

Pull on the ankle and foot to stretch the leg.

Now bend the leg at the knee, supporting the posterior knee and the ankle with your hands, until the foot is flat on the table. Sit on top of the foot and lean your chest into the knee to support the leg. Your goal is to stabilize the leg so that your partner can relax his leg muscles. You now have access to the top of the thigh.

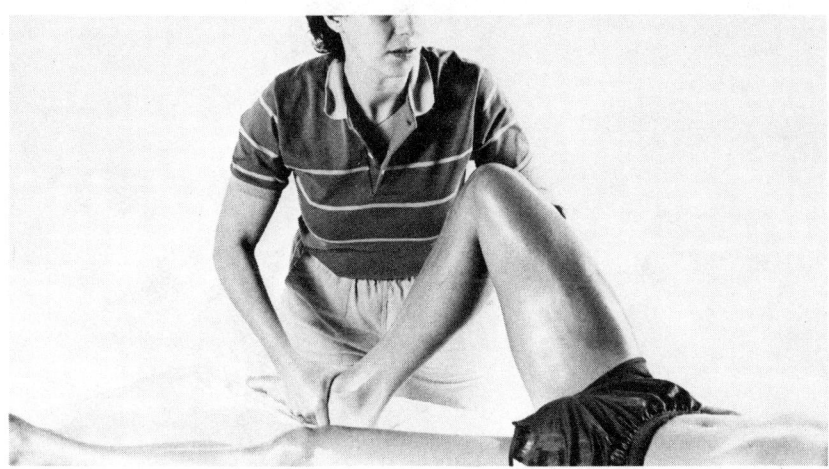

Bend the leg at the knee to relax leg muscles you intend to work.

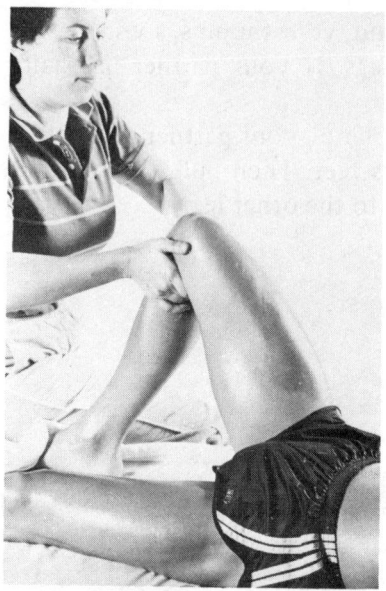

Be sure the foot is flat on the table.

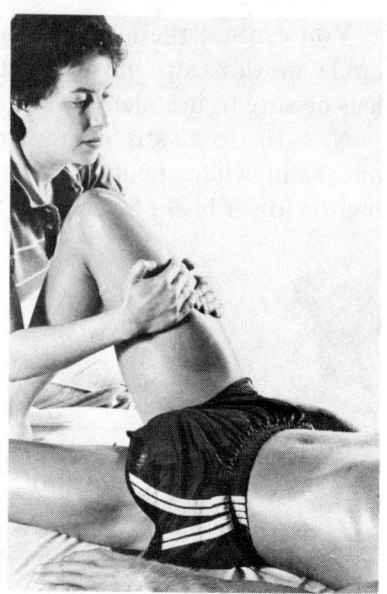

Now you can work the relaxed quadriceps.

Reach to the base of the thigh and with both hands squeeze, pull or lift up to the knee joint.

For the next stroke, you will be pushing on a knee and the opposite shoulder. Stand at your partner's right side. Drape your partner's right leg over his left leg. Place your left hand on his left shoulder and your other hand on his right knee. Now push your arms apart, applying pressure on the shoulder and knee. This

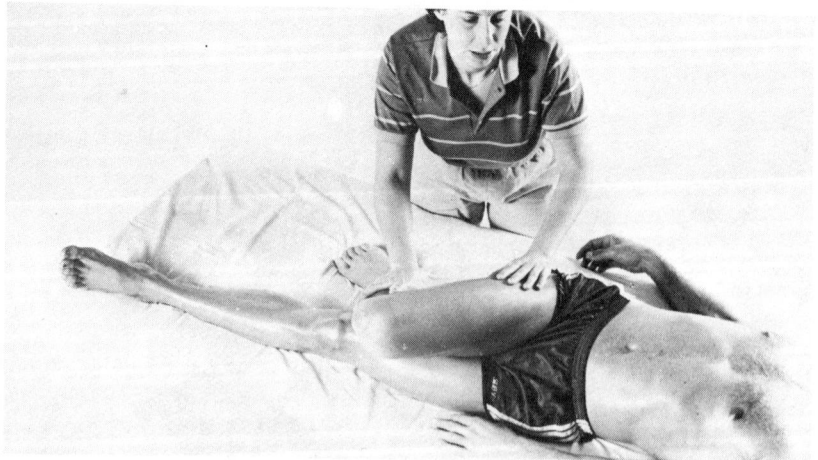

To stretch the hips, drape one leg over another.

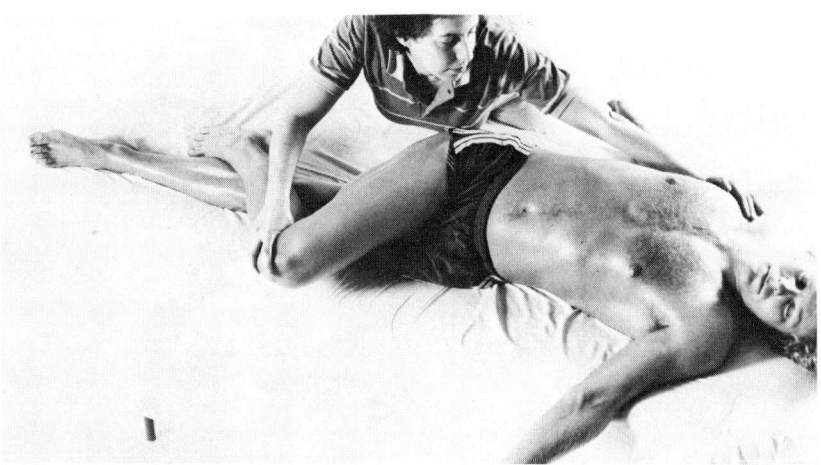

Stretch using your hands.

action stretches the lower back, the iliotibial band and the hips.

You can also stretch the hamstring. Grasp an ankle with one hand and place your other hand under the knee of the same leg. Bend the leg so that your hand is trapped between the hamstring and the calf. Continue bending the leg to stretch the hamstring, by bringing the knee closer to your partner's chest.

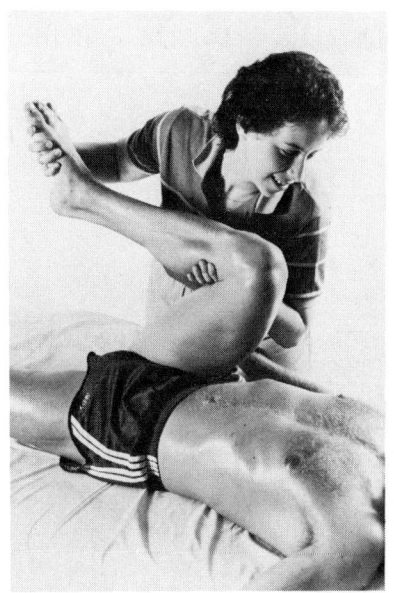

To stretch the hamstrings, hold the foot and bend the knee.

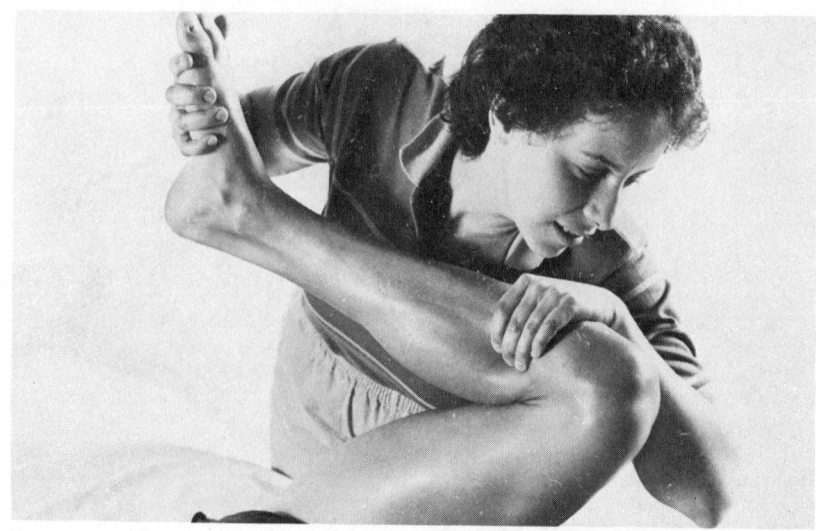

Hold the leg with one hand on the foot, the other hand below the knee.

Finish stretching by working on the Achilles tendon. Stand at the side of the table, near your partner's feet. Place the foot nearest you in the palm of one hand. Anchor the leg above the knee with your other hand. To effect the stretch, pull your forearm toward your body, against the upper foot and toes of your partner. Be sure to keep your hand on the heel of the foot. This stretch affects not only the Achilles tendon, but the foot too.

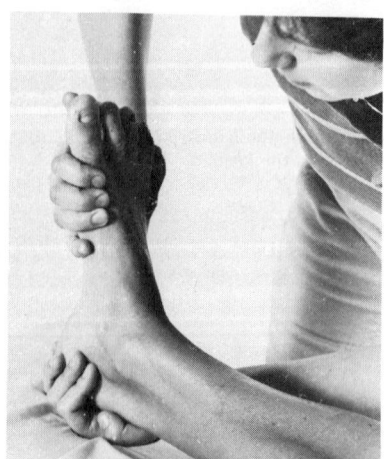

This is one way to stretch the Achilles tendon.

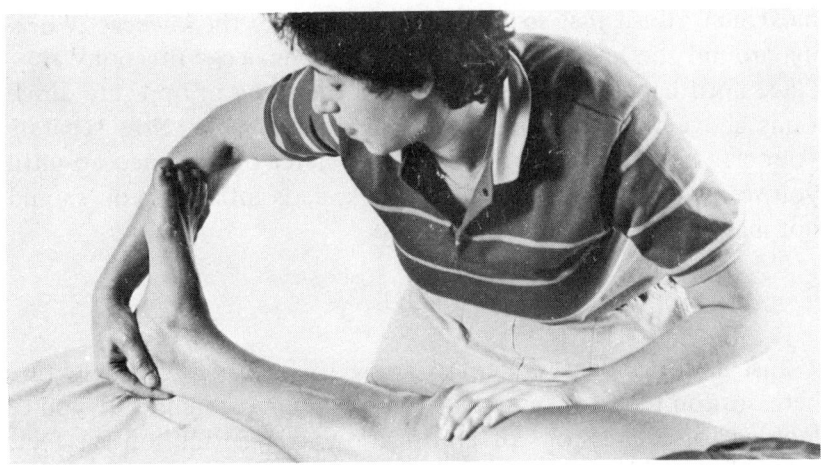

Use the forearm to stretch the Achilles tendon here.

KNEES

From your partner's side you can use a light effleurage stroke to work on a knee. The knee is a complex joint made up of tendons, ligaments, synovial fluid deposits and a large piece of cartilage called the patella, or kneecap. You can feel the kneecap and rotate it gently when the leg is extended, but don't do this as a massage

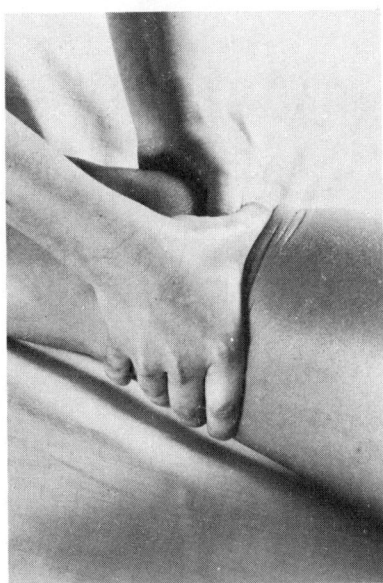

Overlap your thumbs to begin the knee massage.

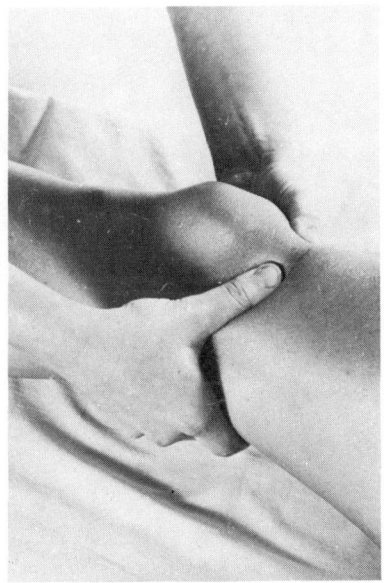

Trace the outline of the kneecap.

movement; do it just so you can get a feel for the kneecap. Working around the kneecap is the best way to massage this bony area. Place both hands, thumbs crossed and pointing in opposite directions above the kneecap, on a thick fold of skin. Now separate your hands and circle around the perimeter of the kneecap until you've made two half-circles. If the knee is inflamed you should not massage it deeply.

FEET

Just about any movement is going to feel excruciatingly fine here so don't be too concerned about your technique. If you're looking for expressions of gratification, concentrate on the feet. Just don't tickle. You might be in the mood to experiment, in which case you should find a reflexology chart. There is a good one in Downing's *The Massage Book.* The chart shows pressure points on the foot that correspond to other parts of the body, which, when worked, are supposed to bring positive effects to that part of the body. You can't hurt your partner if you're careful and he'll enjoy the deep kneading.

Stand at your partner's feet. Now massage each toe, in between the toes and the ridges on the top of the foot. Use one hand to anchor the foot at the heel. Stroke with your first finger between the valleys of the tendons on the top of the foot. Massage each

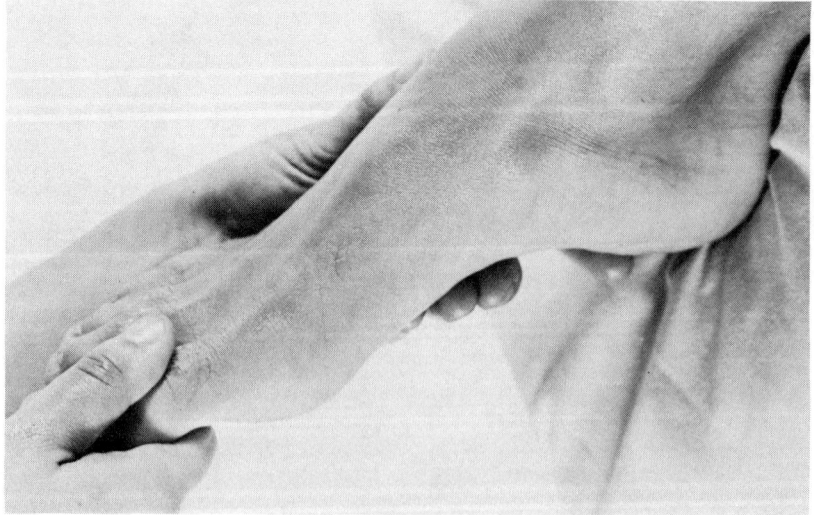

On the foot, work the toes, just like the fingers.

metatarsal, with your thumbs, and the joints of the toes. Massage the arch of the foot. Run the butt of your hand from the toes and down the arch. You can return using that stroke, too. Make a fist and try this stroke. Then use your thumb.

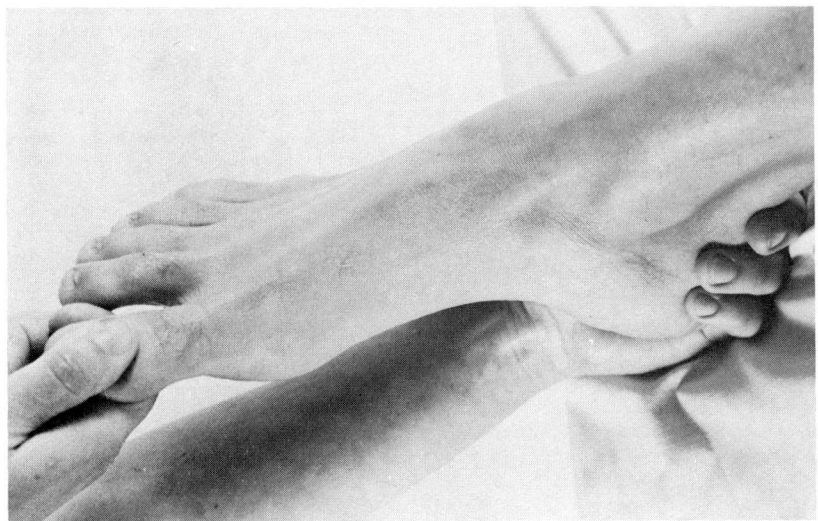

You can anchor the foot at the heel with your hand.

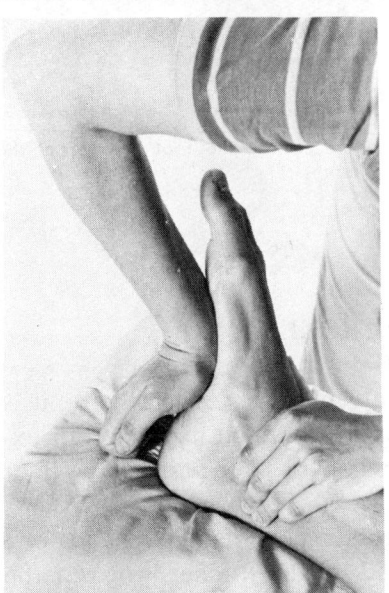

Use the heel of your hand to work the arch of the foot.

Stretching the foot is similar to spreading the hand. Grasp one foot with both hands, fingers together and holding the top of the foot. Put your thumbs together on the metatarsals. Now spread your thumbs, using your fingers as anchors. Stroke to the edge of the foot. Return and repeat the movement.

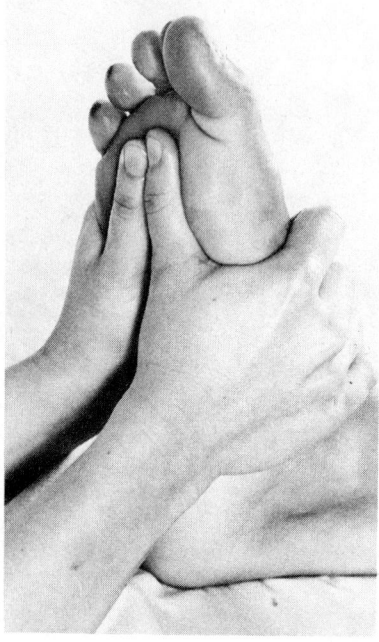

Place your thumbs together to spread the foot.

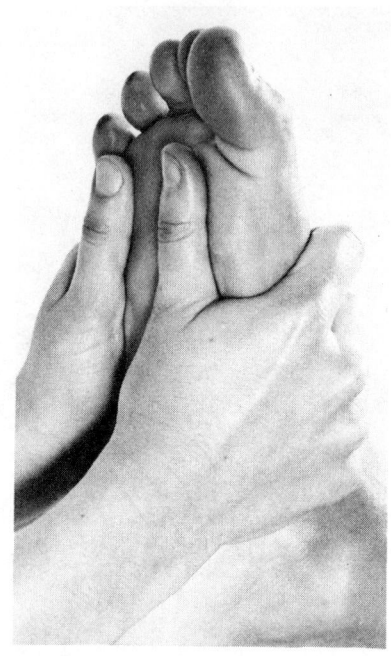

Press against the foot and spread the thumbs.

FINISHING STROKES

Once you have worked the front and back of the body, it is time to finish with some strokes that unify the massage. For example, rest the palms of your hands over your partner's eyes or apply one more very light effleurage stroke over your partner's entire body. You might end by holding the feet or placing one hand on the stomach and one hand on the forehead, or rest the palms of your hands over your partner's eyes. When you're

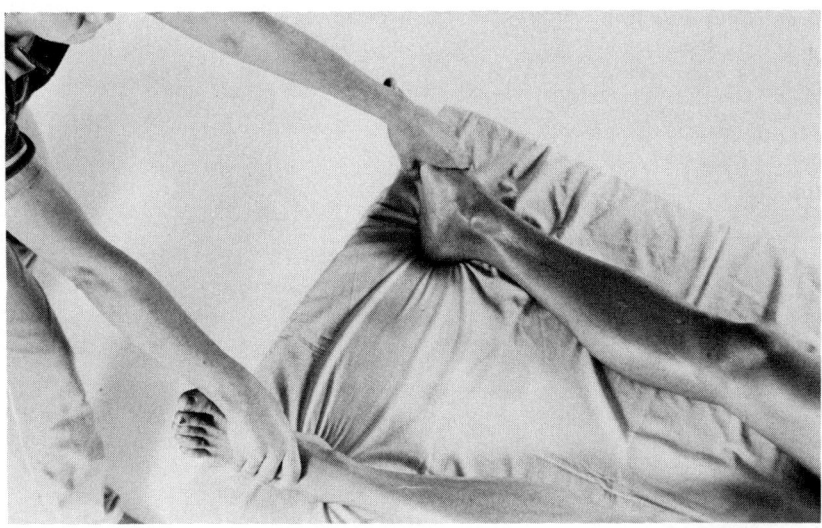

You can finish the massage by holding the ankles.

through, don't disturb your partner. He may have fallen asleep. Cover him with a sheet or blanket and allow him some quiet time alone.

9

Massage for the Young and Elderly

It goes without saying that you're never too old or too young to enjoy or partake in a relaxing massage. While there are a few special rules to consider, the standard massage procedures can be followed without fear of hurting someone, whether he be a one-month-old baby or a man in his seventies. Your greatest barrier is the one the mind puts up—"Oh, he's too old to have a massage; he'll have a heart attack." "Massage your baby. Why you'll get it addicted!" Emotional reactions. And yet often emotions push away logic and common sense, with the result that someone misses out on a pleasurable experience. Massage, when done properly, is no more harmful to your health than spending a day in the sun.

THE YOUNG

There is perhaps not a more enjoyable activity shared between mother and child than a loving caress. A mother needs to hug her child to show her unfathomable love and care. The baby sees the hug, a kiss and a warm breast as a very real reassurance that his new world, away from the protective womb, still carries the vestiges of that security he once knew. A massage merely adds to the bond created between the mother and child. It is food for the infant writes Frederick Leboyer in *Loving Hands*, food as necessary as minerals, vitamins and proteins.

If Leboyer chose to, he could back up his beliefs with an arsenal of data collected from studies on animal behavior. For example, Ashley Montagu writes in *Touching* about an experiment using rats; they are handled gently in infancy. Readings of their serum antibody levels came out higher than other rats not handled so kindly. Higher serum antibody levels indicate that their immunological systems have a much greater resistance to disease. But more importantly, their behavior changed markedly, according to the study: "When handled, the gentled rats were relaxed and yielding. They were not easily frightened. The laboratory attendant had raised them under conditions in which they were frequently handled, stroked and had kindly sounds uttered to them, and they responded with fearlessness, friendliness and a complete lack of neuromuscular tension or irritability. The exact opposite was true of the ungentled rats . . . these animals were frightened and bewildered, anxious and tense."

Apparently, the same factors that influenced rat behavior also apply to people. Continuing studies of the mother-child relationship confirm what we have always sensed through intuition. Mothers who are bonded with their babies in the first hours and days of life later show greater closeness to them, exhibit much more soothing behavior, maintain more eye-to-eye contact and touch their babies more often. Interestingly, these protected and loved children have significantly higher I.Q. scores on the Stanford-Binet test at age 3½ than children who have been separated from their mothers.

During the massage keep in mind that the mother-child bond is established primarily by eye and skin contact and through the mother's soothing voice. By talking softly or humming, the mother creates an atmosphere of calm, which will help relax the baby. A relaxed baby that rests calmly on the mother's legs is much easier to massage than one that flails its arms and legs. Soft background music might also help pacify the child.

The mother will give most of the massages to her baby, but the father can enjoy giving the baby its massage, too. He will gain from the experience just as much as the mother, and the bond between father and child should be strengthened. As is often the case, fathers are pressed for time because of work, while the mother is able to remain at home, when the child is a baby. It is important that the father be sure and set aside plenty of time for giving a massage; the worst thing to do is give a massage when you're rushed. In the event that you have another somewhat older child in the family you might want to let him help with a massage, as well. It might increase the sibling friendship and should the older child harbor any jealousy for want of more attention, allowing him to become involved can reduce this possibility.

Leboyer recommends that you wait a full month after the child's birth before beginning full body massages. Your baby may cry when you begin massaging, but with time he will become accustomed to your actions. You might want to massage him twice a day at first, in the morning and at night before bed. It should take from ten to twenty minutes and don't be surprised if your baby falls asleep by the time you're through massaging. Babies can become just as relaxed from a massage as adults. The age at which you stop massaging your child is a matter of personal choice. Leboyer recommends ending daily massage at six months, when the child can relax on its back. Vimala Schneider, who says she received her inspiration to write *Infant Massage* after meeting Leboyer and seeing baby massage in India, believes that you can continue massaging your children, no matter what their age; of course, you'll probably want to reduce the frequency to once or twice a week. If anything, massage will bring a family closer together.

The mechanics of giving a massage to a baby are the same as with massage for adults. Find a warm room and a pleasant location. In India, the mother places her baby over her outstretched legs. A blanket is draped over her legs to catch any urine the baby might produce. Remember, massage relaxes the entire body. Should you choose this position it would be wise to be able to lean your back against a wall to reduce fatigue. If that position feels uncomfortable, consider just crossing your legs and positioning the baby in front of you on the floor, with a mat under the baby.

A light, natural oil is recommended for baby massage, although if the child's skin is very dry a lotion is advised. Lotions are undesirable otherwise, because they readily soak into the skin and require frequent application. Mrs. Schneider is firmly against using the mass-produced and heavily advertised "baby oils." She says that her research leads her to believe that baby oils contain many toxic substances, which are absorbed into the skin. She not only believes that these oils have no nutritional value, but that they may actually rob the body of vitamins. Leboyer also recommends the use of natural oils, such as almond, olive or coconut.

Where you begin the baby's massage is a matter of choice. But consider starting with the head. Here you can immediately establish eye contact and the baby has the reassurance of your hands being where he can see and feel them. Because your baby has such small dimensions it will often be necessary to use just your fingertips or one hand for massage. The movements you use are almost entirely gentle stroking and bear in mind that a baby is much more susceptible to bruising.

Massage of the appendages can take on a "milking" effect when one of your hands covers an appendage in its entirety. Hold the baby's arm, for example, straight in the air with your left hand. Using your right hand, grasp the baby's arm at the shoulder and gradually bring it up to the baby's hand, where the left hand can then replace the right hand and begin an upward stroke. Repeat this procedure several times. This is the Indian method; the Swedish system recommends a stroking motion from the hand or foot toward the center of the body; however, at this young age, the baby probably isn't going to notice one way or another. Use the stroke you (or your baby) feel most comfortable with.

Massage of the baby's back is crucial because it takes the most stress. Babies spend much of their time on their backs because they are unable to rotate. Begin by placing the baby on its stomach across your outstretched legs. Hold his feet with one hand and slightly elevated. With your free hand begin a long stroke from the neck down to the legs.

The massage would not be complete without a couple of interesting exercises designed to increase the baby's arm and leg coordination. Before the baby is able to walk, it takes the first steps toward that lofty goal by simply flailing with its arms and legs. This prepares him for the effort of walking and improves limb mobility. You can help him along in the following manner. First, start with the arms. The baby should be on its back, with its head pointing away from your body. Grasp both of the baby's hands; your right hand holds his left hand and your left hand holds his right. Now, simultaneously cross the baby's arms. As you make this movement your wrists will uncross. Then return the baby's arms to their original position and repeat this several times. Don't stretch the baby's arms enough to cause discomfort.

The movement is basically the same for the legs. Hold his legs out straight at the ankles and then cross them at the stomach, repeating this motion several times. Each time you should stretch the baby's legs straight. Another movement calls for you to hold your baby's legs at the ankle, then push them, knees bent, up to his tummy. Pull them back straight and repeat several times.

The last movement coordinates the arm and leg. Take his left arm with your right hand and his right leg with your left hand. Now bring his leg up to his ear—that's right, his ear. Babies are extremely flexible so you're not going to hurt him. The arm should be pulled down to his stomach, almost over the extended leg. Repeat several times, switching arms and legs.

You may want to finish the massage session by giving the baby a warm bath.

THE ELDERLY

With age we do not lose our appreciation for the sense of touch. Those who are lucky and have their health will find their final years spent with a loved one. The unlucky will wind up in a "rest home," where a friendly touch is rare.

For now, those elderly who are fortunate enough to be able to receive a massage can rest assured that the methods used for them are no different than for anyone else. There are a few precautions to keep in mind, however. First, your masseur or masseuse shouldn't massage too vigorously. With old age, accumulations of toxic metabolites build up in the system. To throw them suddenly and all at once into the circulatory system places a strain on the body. If the elderly person has never been massaged, begin the massage very gently. Also, the aged tissues are not as elastic as they once were. Their skin is thin and very easily bruised or broken. Be especially careful when kneading so as not to break down the tissue.

Varicose veins are a common problem for the elderly and something to watch for during the massage. It is best to work above a varicose vein at first, by kneading, to create a place where blood can flow when you do work the area around the varicose vein. Use very gentle stroking toward the heart to increase venous drainage.

Dry skin is another common problem with the elderly but that can be easily remedied by using a natural oil for the massage.

With these thoughts in mind you needn't feel hesitant about giving massage to the elderly.

10

Massage for the Athlete

Unfortunately, massage for athletes is a luxury, unless of course you are good enough to be a professional, in which case you have a readily available trainer who can give you a rubdown. This lack of accessibility is unfortunate, because athletes constantly subject their bodies to stress and strain, which results in sore muscles, wrenched knees, ligament strains and general fatigue from endurance competition. Massage can work miracles for all of these debilitating effects. But few athletes take advantage of massage, simply because they cannot afford it. Serious amateur athletes are almost always scraping to get by, especially in sports like cycling and skiing, in which expensive equipment and travel is the rule. In addition, there are few truly professional sports masseurs who make themselves available to the public. The good ones are working for professional sports teams or in private schools and universities.

There is some encouraging news, however. Self-massage is a possibility, which will be described in this chapter and there is a book that will prove most beneficial to the athlete, called *Sportsmassage*. It was written by Jack Meagher, the official masseur for the U.S. Olympic Equestrian Team and Pat Boughton, a writer. Meagher uses Swedish massage and shiatsu in his work and through drawings shows how to massage specific body parts. The book is organized by fifteen specific sports and offers a massage for muscles prone to overuse in each of them.

Some of you who are athletes may still have doubts about the value of massage. The evidence accumulated so far is overwhelmingly favorable, however, and sports massage could be the new frontier to improve performances in many of the minor sports that are just beginning to take advantage of it.

Every professional sport has a trainer who can give massage in one form or another. Ask any professional athlete in the three major sports—baseball, football and basketball—and he'll tell you that he has had a massage to help heal an injury or to work out a muscle spasm. Most often this work is done in the steamy, smelly locker room surrounded by noise, other players and all kinds of medicines and bandages. But massage is so important for one athlete, the boxer, that his trainer is right there at ringside throughout the fight. Between rounds he works his boxer's shoulders, arms and upper back. Without this assistance, the boxer's muscles would tire more easily and his punching would be less crisp and without power. The reason is simple: the trainer is working out the build-up of lactic acid, which causes muscle fatigue.

In another professional sport, cycling, the Europeans have long been receiving leg massage between races. In the stage races, some lasting two weeks, like Tour de France and the Giro de Italia, where there are daily races of up to 150 miles, the legs take incredible punishment and the build-up of lactic acid is inordinate. Were a professional to be without his daily leg massage, he would soon find himself slipping in the standings. Professionals without the benefit of a masseur are never able to win the big races with regularity, the advantage of massage is so crucial.

Finally, runners are the latest of the amateur athletes who are finding that massage can provide the winning formula. They have already gained speed through the use of improved shoes, systematized training regimens, special lightweight nylon clothing, pacing devices such as electronic watches and metronomes, mental preparation, carbohydrate-loading and special diets. The last frontier might just be massage. In East Germany and other Iron Curtain countries massage is a daily convenience for their runners and considering the success of Olympic gold medalist marathoner Waldemar Cierpinski, it must be working.

Recently, Al Salazar, current world-record holder in the marathon with a 2:08:13, a record that stood for twelve years, from 1969 until 1982, revealed that he, too, has been receiving leg massage. Salazar said that deep-tissue massage twice weekly enabled him to maintain, uninterrupted, a seventeen-week training schedule, something he had never been able to accomplish before he started receiving massage. He also attributed the massage with his quick recovery from the world-record performance at the New York City Marathon.

Other forms of bodywork have also gained the interest of athletes. Julius Erving of basketball fame, otherwise known as "Dr. J.," has received private sessions from Moshe Feldenkrais, and Jack Heggie published a book called *Improve Your Skiing*, based on Feldenkrais training methods.

Some forms of bodywork are coming into sportsmedicine, too. Controversy has swirled around Dr. Leroy Perry, a southern California chiropractor who petitioned to join the 1976 Olympic medical team. A chiropractor has never been a member of the U.S. Olympic medical staff and despite a petition signed by over eighty athletes, including several coaches, Perry was denied. Eventually, Perry did go to the Olympics in Montreal, as the head of the Antigua medical committee—an island of 65,000 inhabitants in the Caribbean with an Olympic team of ten members.

Perry treats runners using acupressure. The list of athletes he has treated reads like a who's who: Marty Liquori, Steve Williams, Ken Randle, Clancy Edwards, Dedy Cooper, Russ Hodge, Mike Boit, Dr. Thomas Wessinghage, John Akii-Bua and many more. The problem with Perry is not so much his level of success—it has been noteworthy—but the fact that the medical establishment isn't about to let in "an outsider," who they feel is elbowing in on their turf.

SPORTS AND STRESS AREAS

For those of you who might be considering entering a sports program, you are probably wondering just what part of the body will give you the most pain. This is important if you have a body part that has an inherent weakness or has suffered permanent damage in an accident. Also, some of you may be thinking about switching sports and want to know the pitfalls in a different sport. Every sport has its stresses and strains, some more than others. Here is a partial list of sports and areas to watch out for:

Cycling—posterior, quadriceps, upper back, shoulders, arms, hands, wrists, ankles, back of neck. This is an endurance activity. Leg cramps may result if you ride too far for your condition. Gloves will reduce "road shock" to the hands; "road shock" can

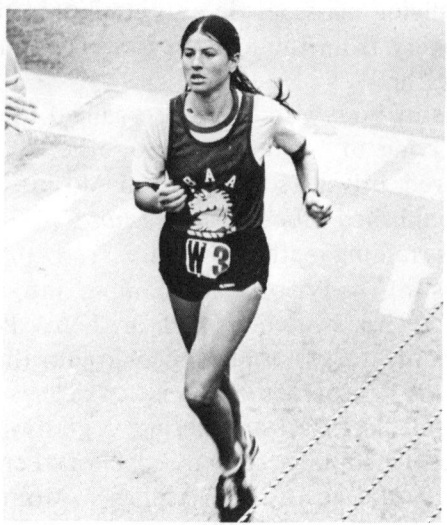

cause numb fingers due to pinching of the ulnar nerve. Sore posteriors result from weak, unused muscles and poorly constructed seats. Do neck exercises during rest stops.

Running—calves, hamstrings, Achilles tendons, shoulders, hips, knees, shins, feet, ankles. This is an endurance activity, unless you are a sprinter. Most of your soreness and injuries will occur below the waist, especially in the knee and hip joints and in the calf and hamstring muscles. Do stretching exercises and build up slowly. Avoid downhill running and uphill running when beginning.

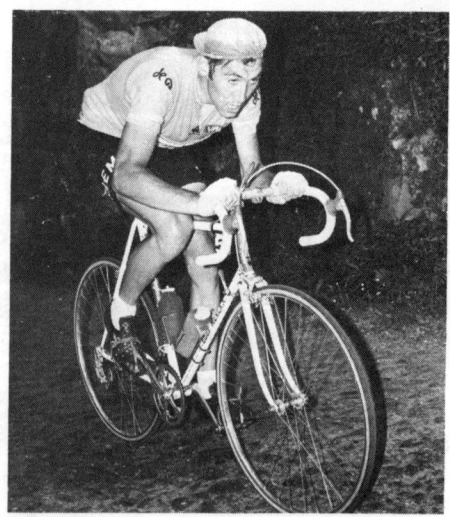

Cross-Country Skiing—ankles, quadriceps, calves, hips, shoulders, arms. This is an endurance activity. Because cross-country skiing is generally a smooth, flowing activity, most of your injuries will occur from overuse or from falling. Your greatest danger is falling and breaking a bone, or pulling a muscle. Torn ligaments are not unheard of. Proper technique will reduce muscle fatigue.

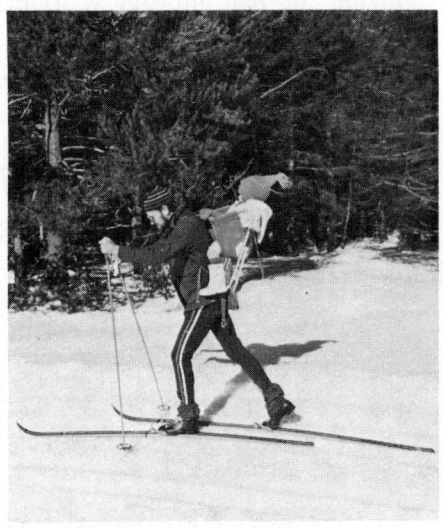

Racquetball or Handball—hands, wrists, waist, arms, elbows, ankles, feet, upper back, shoulders. Much of this sport is anaerobic in competitive situations. The danger here is with twisting

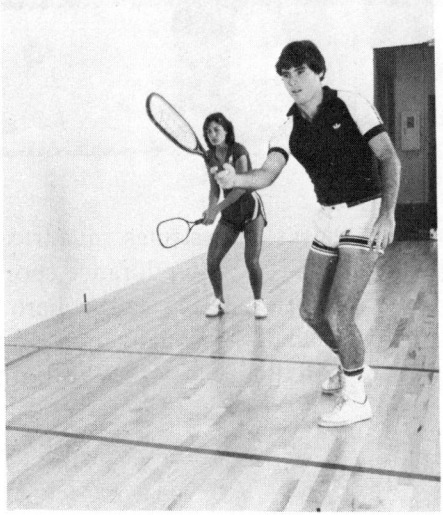

too quickly to reach the ball and straining a muscle. In handball there is a very real danger of damaging the circulatory system in the hands. Racquetball players sometimes develop "tennis elbow."

Tennis—elbows, arms, shoulders, upper back, lower back, knees, hamstrings, hips. This is an endurance activity, with some anaerobic effort required. The big problem is "tennis elbow," an injury caused by hitting the ball improperly. It primarily affects the extensor muscles of the forearm and tendons surrounding the elbow joint. Lunging for the ball can cause ankle strains and pulled muscles.

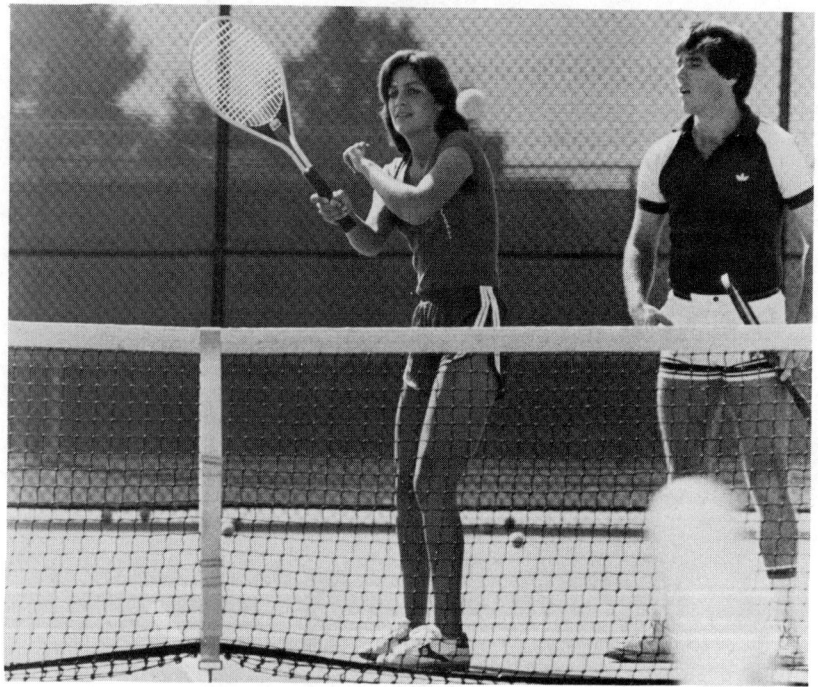

Soccer—shins, feet, calves, hamstrings, quadriceps, lower and upper back, hips, head. This is an endurance sport that calls for considerable anaerobic effort. The big danger here is being kicked or falling when hitting the ball. Although a non-contact sport, two bodies have a way of colliding when they're both aiming for a single object, the ball.

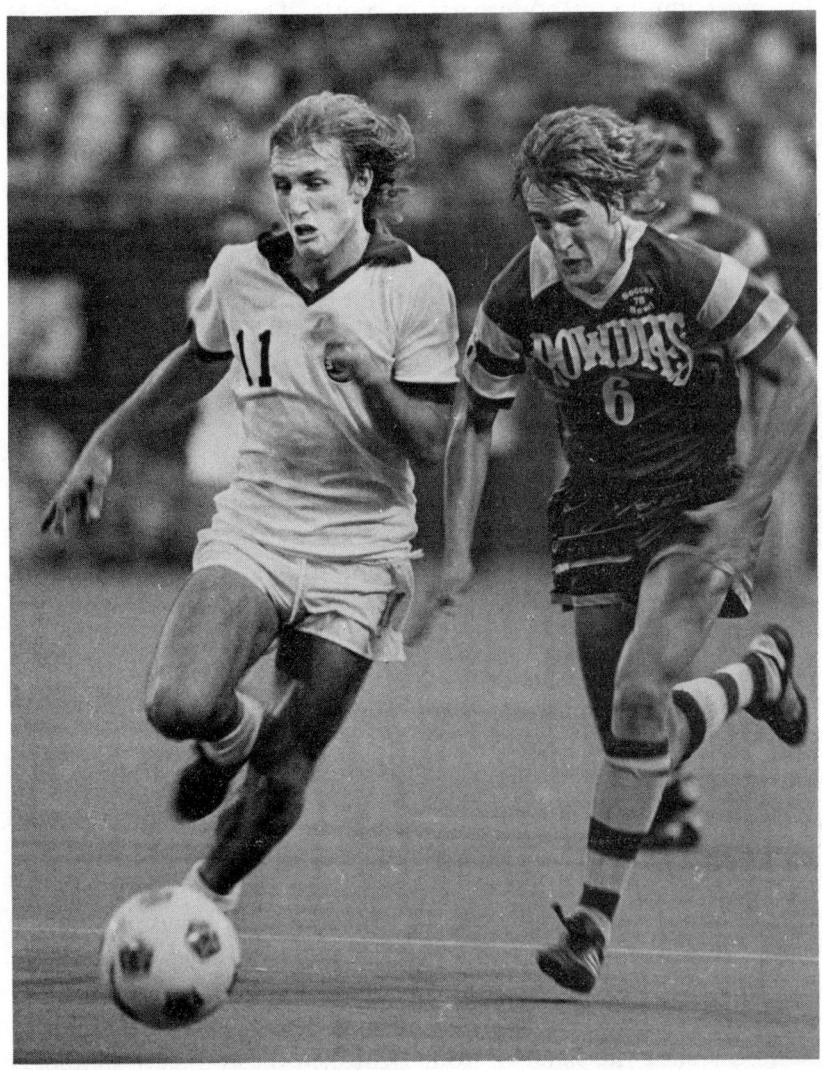

SELF-MASSAGE TECHNIQUES

Giving yourself a massage isn't the easiest thing to do, although it can be accomplished on some parts of the body and will provide limited benefits. Touching yourself doesn't have the same power as having someone else work on your body, but many of the circulatory benefits can still be gained.

Fortunately, the legs are readily accessible and they are perhaps the most important body parts in sports. There are two positions from which you can massage your legs comfortably and effectively. Sit down on the floor, with one leg bent at the knee and the other one extended. First stroke the calf and then the hamstring on the bent leg. Always stroke up toward your heart. Beginning at the ankle, wrap your thumbs behind the lower calf. Your fingers will follow the ridge of your shin. Now bring the hands up together, pushing your thumbs against your calf muscle. Now reverse your hand position. Begin again at the ankle. Place your fingers on the calf and your thumbs on the ridge of the shin. Bring your hands up simultaneously as far as the knee. Using this stroke, continue up the hamstring. Your hands will separate before reaching your hip.

To improve venous drainage assume this position: lean back against a couch near a wall and prop one leg up against the wall. Now you can use a hand stroke for the legs, thumbs following the ridge of your shin, fingers working the calf and hamstring.

Neck massage is easy to do for yourself and very relaxing. Lie on your back on the floor. A bed is usually too soft. Now bring your hands to the back of your neck. Push your head back and forth using your hands. Be gentle and do not force the neck. This is a good procedure for those with whiplash. Rocking your neck back and forth without pain tells the neural patterns that it can move freely. You can also position your hands on the sides of your face or the jaw for better leverage if you have a very stiff neck.

A final note about how to get up from the floor, especially for those with bad necks. Getting up can be stressful if not done properly, and will take away everything you have gained from doing the exercises while lying on your back. Here is the proper method: place the hand of your right arm on your left shoulder. Now roll onto your left side. (Place the hand of your left arm on your right shoulder and roll onto your right side if you prefer getting up on your right side.) Put your right hand on the floor, next to your left shoulder. Use your right arm now to push yourself up. Let your neck hang down to your chin. Your arm is doing all the work, not your neck. As you straighten your right arm, bring your left arm to your left side and also push off the floor with it. Now swing your body straight, at the waist, and use your legs to do the rest of the work of getting onto your feet. Your neck has been saved from unnecessary stress.

Glossary

ABDUCTION–The lateral movement of the limbs *away* from the median plane of the body; to draw away from the median plane of the body.

ABDUCTOR POLLICIS BREVIS–Muscle that abducts the thumb. Origin is ridge of trapezium and transverse carpal ligament. Insertion is outer side of first phalanx of thumb.

ABDUCTOR DIGITI QUINTI–Muscle that abducts little finger. Origin is pisiform bone and ligaments. Insertion is inner side of first phalanx of little finger.

ACHILLES TENDON–The tendon of the gastrocnemius and soleus muscles of the leg.

ADDUCTION–Movement of a limb *toward* the median plane of the body.

ADDUCTOR BREVIS–Muscle that flexes and adducts the thigh. Origin is the ramus of pubis. Insertion is the femur.

ADDUCTOR LONGUS–Muscle that adducts and flexes the thigh. Origin is the pubic crest and insertion is the femur.

ADDUCTOR MAGNUS–Muscle that adducts the thigh and rotates it outward. Origin is the pubis and insertion is the femur.

APONEUROSIS–A flat, fibrous sheet of connective tissue that serves to attach muscle to bone or other tissue. May sometimes serve as fascia.

ARTERY–One of the vessels carrying blood from the heart to the tissues. The arteries carry the oxygenated blood from the right and left ventricles of the heart to all parts of the body.

ARTICULATE–To join together as a joint.

ARTICULATION–The place or union between two or more bones; a joint. It is classified as being immovable (synarthrosis), slightly movable (amphiarthrosis), or freely movable (diathrosis).

BICEPS BRACHII—Muscle that flexes the arm and forearm and supinates the hand. Origin is the scapula and insertion is the radius.

BICEPS FEMORIS—Muscle that flexes the knee and rotates it outward. Origin is the short head from linea aspera and long head from ischial tuberosity. Insertion is the head of the fibula lateral condyle of the tibia.

BRACHIALIS—Muscle that flexes the forearm. Origin is the lower half of the anterior surface of the humerus and insertion is at the ulna.

BRACHIORADIALIS—Muscle that flexes and supinates the forearm.

CALCANEUM—Also known as calcaneus. The heel bone, or os calcis. It articulates with the cuboid bone and with the astragalus.

CAPILLARIES—Any of the minute blood vessels, averaging .008 mm in diameter, carrying blood and forming the capillary system. Capillaries connect the smallest arteries (arterioles) with the smallest veins (venules).

CERVICAL VERTEBRAE—First seven bones of the spinal column.

CLAVICLE—The collarbone; the bone that articulates with the sternum and the scapula.

COCCYX—Small bone at the base of the spinal column, formed by four fused rudimentary vertebrae.

CONDYLE—A rounded protuberance at the end of a bone forming an articulation.

CUBOID BONE—Outer bone of the tarsal or instep bones articulating posteriorly with the fourth and fifth metatarsus.

CUNEIFORM BONES—Those of the internal, middle, and external tarsus.

DELTOIDEUS—Muscle that raises the arm and rotates. Origin is the clavicle and insertion is the shaft of the humerus.

DIGASTRICUS—Muscle consisting of the anterior and posterior bellies. Draws hyoid bone forward and backward. Origin is lower border of lower jaw and insertion is intermediate tendon between both bellies.

DISTAL PHALANX—The toe or finger bone most remote from the metacarpus or metatarsus.

EPIDERMIS–Cuticle, or outer layer of skin. It is formed from within outward. It consists of four layers or strata.

EXTENSOR CARPI RADIALIS LONGUS–Muscle that extends and abducts the wrist. Origin is the humerus and insertion is the base of the second metacarpal.

EXTENSOR DIGITORUM LONGUS–Muscle that extends the toes and flexes the foot. Origin is the external tuberosity of the tibia and insertion is the second and third phalanges of the toes.

FEMUR–The thigh bone. It extends from the hip to the knee and is the longest and strongest bone in the skeleton.

FIBULA–The outer and smaller bone of the leg from the ankle to the knee, articulating above with the tibia and below with the tibia and talus. One of the longest and thinnest bones of the skeleton.

FLEXOR CARPI RADIALIS–Muscle that consists of humeral head and ulnar head. It flexes and adducts the wrist. Origin is the humerus and insertion is the metacarpal.

FLEXOR CARPI ULNARIS–Muscle consists of humeral head and ulnar head. It flexes and adducts wrist. Origin is humerus and insertion is pisiform bone and fifth metacarpal.

FLEXOR DIGITI QUINTI BREVIS–Muscle flexes first phalanx of little finger. Origin is unciform bone and insertion is first phalanx of little finger.

FLEXOR DIGITORUM ACCESSORIUS–Muscle that assists flexing of the toes. Origin is the inferior surface of os calcis by two heads from outer and inner bones. Insertion is tendons of flexor digitorum longus.

FLEXOR DIGITORUM BREVIS–Muscle that flexes the toes. Origin is plantar fascia and insertion is the second phalanges of lesser toes.

FLEXOR DIGITORUM LONGUS–Muscle that flexes phalanges and extends toes. Origin is the lower portion of the shaft of fibula and insertion is the distal phalanx of the great toe.

FLEXOR DIGITORUM SUPERFICIALIS–Muscle that consists of three heads: humeral, ulnar and radial. It flexes the middle phalanges and hand. Origin is the humerus, medial side of coronoid process and outer border of radius. Insertion is second phalanx of each finger.

FLEXOR HALLUCIS BREVIS—Muscle that flexes the great toe. Origin is the internal surface of cuboid and middle and external cuneiform bones and insertion is at the sides of the base of the first phalanx of the great toe.

FLEXOR HALLUCIS LONGUS—Muscle that flexes the great toe and extends the foot. Origin is the lower portion of the fibula and insertion is the distal phalanx of the great toe.

FLEXOR POLLICIS BREVIS—Muscle flexes first phalanx of thumb. Origin is transverse carpal ligament and metacarpal bone. Insertion is base of first phalanx of thumb.

FLEXOR POLLICIS LONGUS—Muscle that flexes the thumb. origin is the anterior surface of the middle third of radius and insertion is the terminal phalanx of thumb.

FRONTAL—The forehead bone.

FRONTAL FONTANEL—Opposite location of the occipital fontanel.

GASTROCNEMIUS—Muscle that flexes the foot and leg. Origin is the external and internal femoral condyles. Insertion is into os calcis.

GLUTEUS MAXIMUS—Muscle that extends and rotates the thigh. Origin is the superior curved iliac line and crest and coccyx and sacrum. Insertion is fascia lata and the femur below greater trochanter.

GLUTEUS MEDIUS—Muscle that abducts and rotates the thigh. Origin is the lateral surface of the ilium. Insertion is the greater trochanter.

GLUTEUS MINIMUS—Muscle that abducts and extends the thigh. Origin is the lateral surface of the ilium. Insertion is the greater trochanter.

GRACILIS—Muscle that flexes and adducts the leg; adducts the thigh. Origin is the pubis and insertion is the tibia.

HUMERUS—Upper bone of the arm from the elbow to the shoulder joint, where it articulates with the scapula.

HYOID BONE—Horseshoe-shaped bone at the base of the tongue.

ILLIAC CREST—The hip.

ILIOCOSTALIS CERVICIS—Muscle that extends the cervical spine. Origin is angles of third and sixth ribs and insertion is transverse processes of fourth and sixth cervical vertebrae.

ILIOCOSTALIS THORACIS—Muscle that keeps the dorsal spine erect. Origin is the angles of twelfth and seventh ribs and insertion is the sixth to first ribs and seventh cervical vertebra.

ILLIACUS—This muscle flexes and rotates the thigh. Origin is the iliac fossa and insertion is the lesser trochanter.

ILIOCOSTALIS LUMBORUM—Muscle that extends the lumbar spine. Origin is with sacrospinalis. Insertion is in angles of fifth to twelfth ribs.

INSERTION—The manner or place of attachment of a muscle to the bone so that it moves.

INTERCOSTALES—(internal and external) Muscles that draw ribs together and lower ribs. Origin is the lower border of the rib and insertion is the upper border of the rib below.

INTERTRANSVERSARLI—Muscle that flexes the vertebral column. Origin is between transverse processes of contiguous vertebrae.

ISCHIUM—Lower portion of the hip bone.

KNEADING—A form of massage consisting of grasping, wringing, lifting, rolling or pressing part of a muscle or group of muscles.

LATISSIMUS DORSI—Muscle that adducts, extends and rotates the arm. Origin is the lower thoracic and lumbar vertebrae and insertion is the humerus.

LEVATOR SCAPULAE—Muscle that elevates the posterior angle of the scapula. Origin is the transverse processes of four upper cervical vertebrae and insertion is the scapula.

LEVATORES COSTARUM—Muscle that raises ribs and flexes vertebral column. Origin is the transverse process of the seventh cervical and upper eleven thoracic vertebrae. Insertion is the rib next below.

LIGAMENT—A band or sheet of strong fibrous connective tissue connecting the articular ends of bones serving to bind them together and to facilitate or limit motion.

LONGISSIMUS CERVICIS—Muscle that extends the cervical spine. Origin is the upper thoracic vertebrae and insertion is the ribs and lumbar and dorsal vertebrae.

LONGISSIMUS THORACIS—Muscle that extends the spinal column. Origin is the transverse process of the lumbar and dorsal vertebrae and insertion is the lowest ribs and lumbar and dorsal vertebrae.

LUMBAR VERTEBRAE—The five vertebrae between the thoracic vertebrae and the sacrum.

LYMPHATIC SYSTEM—That system involved in the conveyance of lymph from the tissues to the bloodstream. It includes the lymph capillaries, lacteals, lymph nodes, lymph vessels and main lymph ducts.

LYMPH NODE—A rounded body consisting of accumulations of lymphatic tissue found at intervals in the course of lymphatic vessels. Lymph nodes vary in size from a pinhead to an olive and may occur singly or in groups. Lymph nodes act as filters, keeping particulate matter, especially bacteria, from getting into the bloodstream.

MANDIBLE—The horseshoe-shaped bone forming the lower jaw.

MASSAGE—From the Greek word to knead. Manipulation, methodical pressure, friction and kneading of the body. Normally applied upon the bare skin.

MASSEUR—A man who gives massage.

MASSEUSE—A woman who gives massage.

MASTOID PROCESS—Nipple-shaped process of mastoid portion of temporal bone that lies behind the external opening of the ear and below the temporal line. Serves for attachment of sternocleidomastoid.

MAXILLARY—Relating to the upper jaw.

METACARPAL—Pertaining to the bones of the metacarpus or bones of the hand.

MIDDLE PHALANX—The phalanx (where there are three) intermediate between distal and priximal phalanges.

MYLOHYOIDEUS—Muscle that elevates the floor of the mouth and hyoid and depresses the jaw. Origin is the mandible and insertion is body of hyoid.

NASAL—Relating to the nose.

NAVICULAR—Scaphoid bones in the carpus (wrist) and in the tarsus (ankle).

NERVE—A bundle or a group of bundles of nerve fibers outside the central nervous system that connect the brain and spinal cord with various parts of the body. Nerves conduct afferent impulses centrally from receptor organs and efferent impulses peripherally to effector tissues and organs.

OBLIQUUS EXTERNUS ABDOMINIS—Muscle that contracts the abdomen and viscera. Origin is the lower eight ribs and insertion is the iliac crest.

OBLIQUUS INTERNUS ABDOMINIS—Muscle that compresses viscera, and flexes thorax forward. Origin is the iliac crest and insertion is the few lowest ribs.

OCCIPITAL BONE—Bone in lower back portion of skull between the parietal and temporal bones.

OCCIPITAL FONTANEL—An unossified space or soft spot lying between the cranial bones of the skull of a fetus in the back portion of the head.

OMOHYOIDEUS—Muscle that depresses the hyoid. Origin is the upper border of the scapula and insertion is the hyoid bone.

OPPONENS DIGITI QUINTI—Muscle flexes and adducts little finger. Origin is unciform bone and insertion is fifth metacarpal bone.

ORBIT—The bony pyramid-shaped cavity of the skull that contains and protects the eyeballs.

ORIGIN—The more fixed attachment of a muscle; the source of the muscle.

PALMARIS LONGUS—Muscle that tightens palmar fascia, flexes the wrist. Origin is the humerus and insertion is the transverse carpal ligament and palmar fascia.

PARIETAL BONE—One of two bones that together form the roof and sides of the skull.

PATELLA—A lens-shaped bone situated in front of the knee in the tendon of the quadriceps femoris muscle. Also known as the kneecap.

PECTINEUS—Muscle that flexes and adducts the thigh. Origin is the pubic spine and insertion is the pectineal line of the femur.

PECTORALIS MAJOR—Muscle that flexes, adducts and rotates the arm. Origin is the sternum and insertion is the humerus.

PELVIC GIRDLE—Arch made by the innominate (nameless) bones.

PEROISTIUM—The fibrous membrane that forms the investing covering of bones except at their articular surfaces. Peroistium serves as a supporting structure for blood vessels nourishing bone and for attachment of muscles, tendons and ligaments.

PERONEUS BREVIS—The muscle that extends and abducts the foot. Origin is the midportion of the shaft of the fibula. Insertion is the base of the fifth metatarsal bone.

PERONEUS LONGUS—Muscle that extends, abducts and everts

the foot. Origin is the upper fibula and external condyle of the tibia. Insertion is by tendon to internal cuneiform and first metatarsal bone.

PERONEUS TERTIUS—Muscle that flexes the foot. Origin is the lower part of the fibula. Insertion is the fifth metatarsal bone.

PLANTARIS—Muscle that extends foot. Origin is the femur and insertion is the inner border of the tendo calcaneus.

POPLITEUS—Muscle that flexes the leg and rotates it inward. Origin is the femur and insertion is the tibia.

PRONATOR TERES—Muscle that consists of the humeral head and the ulnar head and works to pronate the hand. Origin is the humerus and insertion is the radius.

PROXIMAL PHALANX—The toe or finger bone that articulates with a metacarpal or metatarsal bone.

PSOAS MAJOR—Muscle that flexes the thigh, adducts and rotates it medially. Origin is the last thoracic and all of the lumbar vertebrae and insertion is the femur.

PSOAS MINOR—Muscle that tenses the iliac fascia. Origin is the twelfth thoracic and first lumbar vertebrae. Insertion is the iliac fascia.

QUADRATE—Square, or having four equal sides.

QUADRATUS LUMBORUM—Muscle that flexes the trunk laterally and forward. Origin is the iliac crest and insertion is the twelfth rib and the upper lumbar vertebrae.

RADIUS—The outer and shorter bone of the arm that revolves partially about the ulna.

RAMUS—Branch. One of the divisions of a forked structure.

RECTUS ABDOMINIS—Muscle that compresses the abdomen. Origin is the pubis and insertion is the cartilage of fifth to seventh ribs.

RECTUS FEMORIS—Muscle that extends the leg. Origin is the iliac spine and insertion is the base of the patella.

RHOMBOIDEUS—One of two muscles beneath the trapezius muscle. Origin is the spinous processes of the second to fifth thoracic vertebrae and insertion is the vertebral border of the scapula below the spine (for rhomboideus major).

RIB—One of a series of 12 pairs of narrow, curved bones extending laterally and anteriorly from sides of thoracic vertebrae. With the exception of the floating ribs, they are connected to the sternum by means of costal cartilages.

SACRUM—Formed of five united vertebrae, it makes up the base of the vertebral column and. with the coccyx, forms the posterior boundary of the true pelvis. The sacrum in a male is narrower and more curved than in a female.

SCALENUS ANTERIOR—The muscle that elevates the first rib and flexes the neck. Its origin is the third to sixth cervical vertebrae and its insertion is the tubercle of the first rib.

SCALENUS POSTERIOR—The muscle that elevates the second rib and flexes the neck. Its origin is the fourth to sixth cervical vertebrae and its insertion is the second rib.

SCAPHOID—A proximal boat-shaped bone of the carpus or the tarsus.

SCAPULA—The large, flat, triangular bone that forms the posterior part of the shoulder. It articulates with the clavicle and the humerus.

SEMIMEMBRANOSUS—Muscle that flexes and rotates the leg and extends the thigh. Origin is the ischial tuberosity and insertion is the medial condyle of the tibia.

SEMISPINALIS CAPITIS—Muscle that rotates and draws the head backward. Origin is the transverse processes of the upper six or seven thoracic and lower four cervical vertebrae. Insertion is the occipital bone.

SEMISPINALIS THORACIS—Muscle that erects the vertebral column. Origin is the transverse processes of the sixth to tenth thoracic vertebrae. Insertion is the spines of the upper four thoracic and lower two cervical vertebrae.

SEMITENDINOSUS—Muscle that flexes and rotates the leg and extends the thigh. Origin is the ischial tuberosity and insertion is the shaft of the tibia below the internal tuberosity.

SERRATUS ANTERIOR—Muscle that elevates the ribs and rotates the scapula. Origin is the upper eight or nine ribs. Insertion is the angles and vertebral border of the scapula.

SOLEUS—Muscle that extends and rotates the foot. Origin is the upper shaft of the fibula and insertion is by tendo calcaneus to os calcis.

SPINALIS THORACIS—Muscle that erects the spinal column. Origin is the spines of the first two lumbar and last two thoracic vertebrae. Insertion is the spines of middle and upper thoracic vertebrae.

SPLENIUS CAPITIS—Muscle that rotates and extends the head. Origin is the spines of third and sixth thoracic vertebrae and insertion is the transverse processes of the first and second cervical vertebrae.

STERNOCLEIDOMASTOIDEUS—The muscle that rotates and depresses the head. It originates in the sternum and clavicle and inserts at the mastoid process.

STERNOHYOIDEUS—Depresses hyoid bone. Origin is the manubrium sterni and insertion is the body of hyoid bone.

STERNOTHYREOIDEUS—Muscle that depresses the thyroid cartilage. Origin is the sternum and insertion is the side of thyroid cartilage.

STERNUM—The narrow, flat bone in the median line of the thorax in front. It consists of three portions distinguished as the manubrium, the gladiolus and the ensiform of xiphoid process.

STYLOHYOIDEUS—Muscle that elevates and dilates the pharynx. Origin is the styloid process and insertion is the thyroid cartilage and side of pharynx.

TALUS—The ankle bone articulating with the tibia, fibula, calcaneus and navicular bone.

TEMPORAL—Relating to the temples of the head.

TEMPORALIS MASSETER—The muscle that closes the mouth and is the principle muscle in mastication.

TENDON—Fibrous connective tissue serving for the attachment of muscles to bones and other parts.

THORACIC VERTEBRAE—The 12 vertebrae that connect the ribs and form part of the posterior wall of the thorax.

THYREOHYOIDEUS—Muscle that depresses the hyoid bone; elevates thyroid cartilage if hyoid bone is fixed. Origin is the side of thyroid cartilage and insertion is cornu and body of hyoid bone.

TIBIA—The inner and larger bone of the leg between the knee and ankle articulating with the femur above and with the talus below.

TIBIALIS ANTERIOR—Muscle that elevates and flexes the foot. Origin is the upper tibia and insertion is the internal cuneiform and first metatarsal.

TIBIALIS POSTERIOR—Muscle that extends tarsus and inverts the foot. Origin is the shaft of fibula and tibia and insertion is the second to fourth metatarsal.

TRAPEZIUS--This muscle draws the head back and to the side and rotates the scapula. Origin is the thoracic vertebrae and it inserts at the clavicle.

TRICEPS BRACHII--Muscle that extends forearm and arm. Origin is the scapula and humerus and insertion is the ulna.

TROCHANTER--Either of the two bony processes below the neck of the femur.

TUBEROSITY--An elevated round process of a bone.

ULNA--The inner and larger bone of the forearm, between the wrist and the elbow, on the side opposite that of the thumb.

VASTUS LATERALIS--Muscle that extends the knee. Origin is the trochanter and insertion is tendons of quadriceps femoris.

VASTUS MEDIALIS--Muscle that extends the leg; it draws the patella in. Origin is the femur and insertion is the common tendon of quadriceps femoris.

VEIN--Vessel carrying dark red (unaerated) blood to the heart, except for the pulmonary vein, which carries oxygenated blood. Veins have three coats: inner, middle, and outer.

VISCERA--Internal organs enclosed within a cavity, especially the abdominal organs.

ZYGOMATIC PROCESS--A thin projection from the temporal bone bounding its scale-like portion.

Bibliography

Berkson, Devaki. *The Foot Book*. New York: Funk and Wagnalls, 1977.

Downing, George. *The Massage Book*. New York: Randon House, 1972.

Duke, Marc. *Acupuncture*. New York: Pyramid Communications, Inc., 1972.

Feitis, Rosemary, ed. *Ida Rolf Talks About Rolfing and Physical Reality*. New York: Harper and Row, 1978.

Fox, Charles. "The Feldenkrais Phenomenon." *Quest/80*, December/January 1978.

Glover, T.R. *From Pericles to Philip*. 3rd ed. London: Methaen and Company Ltd., 1917.

Gray, Henry. *Gray's Anatomy*, ed. T. Pickering Pick and Robert Howden, New York: Crown Publishers, 1901.

Inkeles, Gordon, and Murray Todris. *The Art of Sensual Massage*. New York: Simon and Schuster, 1972.

Johnson, Clive. "An Interview with John Thie, D.C." *Science of Mind*. Sept. 1977.

Kellogg, John Harvey. *The Art of Massage*. Milwaukee: C.N. Casper Co., 1929 rev.

Krusen, Frank H. *Physical Medicine*. Philadelphia: W.B. Saunders Company, 1941.

Leboyer, Frederick. *Loving Hands*. New York: Alfred A. Knopf, Inc., 1976.

Manaka, Yoshio, and Ian Urquhart. *The Layman's Guide to Acupuncture*. New York: John Weatherhill, Inc., 1972.

Mann, Edward W. *Orgone, Reich and Eros*. New York: Simon and Schuster, 1973.

Meagher, Jack, and Pat Boughton. *Sportsmassage*. New York: Dolphin Books Doubleday and Company, 1980.

Monkerud, Donald. "All Medicine Has a Place in Sports." *On the Run*, December 21, 1978, pp. 12-15.

Namikoshi, Tokujiro. *Shiatsu*. Tokyo: Japan Publications, 1969.

Nissen, Hartvig. *Practical Massage and Corrective Exercises With Applied Anatomy*. Philadelphia: F.A. Davis Company, 1929 rev.

Ostrenga, Linda. *Healthsource: A Guide to Humanistic & Holistic Health Resources on the Peninsula*. Menlo Park, Calif: Linda Ostrenga, 1980.

Palmer, Margaret. *Lessons on Massage*. 6th ed. London: Bailliere, Tindall and Cox, 1927.

Rolf, Ida P. *Rolfing—The Integration of Human Structures*. Santa Monica, Calif.: Dennis Landman Publishers, 1977.

Rosenfeld, Albert. "Teaching the Body How to Program the Brain is Moshe's Miracle." *Smithsonian Magazine*, January 1982, pp. 53-58.

Schneider, Vimala. *Infant Massage—A Handbook for Loving Parents*. Aurora, Colo., Vimala Schneider, 1979.

Segal, Maybelle. *Reflexology*. North Hollywood, Calif.: Hal Leighton Printing Co., 1976.

Shestack, Robert. *Handbook of Physical Therapy*. New York: Springer Publishing, 1956.

Taber, Clarence Wilbur. *Taber's Cyclopedic Medical Dictionary*, ed. Clayton L. Thomas. Philadelphia: F.A. Davis Co., 1940.

Tappan, Frances M. *Healing Massage Techniques—A Study of Eastern and Western Methods*. Reston, Va.: Reston Publishing Company, 1980.

Teeguarden, Iona. *Acupressure Way of Health*. San Francisco: Japan Publications, 1978.

Thie, John F. *Touch for Health*. Marina del Rey, Calif.: DeVorss & Company, 1979.

Whittaker, Peter. *The American Way of Sex*. New York: G.P. Putnam's Sons, 1974.

Wischnia, Bob. "Rolfing." *Runner's World*, January 1979, pp. 76-81.

Wolf, Heinrich F. *Textbook of Physical Therapy*. New York: D. Appleton-Century Company, 1933.

Wood, Elizabeth, and Paul D. Becker. *Beard's Massage, Principles and Techniques,* 3rd ed. Philadelphia: W.B. Saunders Company, 1980.

About The Author

Ray Hosler is the senior editor of *Runner's World* Books. He has also been an editor with *Runner's World* magazine and with two daily newspapers. He earned his bachelor's degree in Technical Journalism from Colorado State University. Because of a recent accident that left him with whiplash and numerous muscle imbalances, he became interested in bodywork and massage, which culminated in this, his first book.

Recommended Reading

The following books, also available from Anderson World, can augment your exercise and fitness program. They are available from major bookstores or can be ordered directly from the publisher (1400 Stierlin Road, Mountain View, CA 94043).

RUNNER'S WORLD YOGA BOOK by Jean Couch with Nell Weaver. An easy-to-follow guide to using the principles of yoga for stretching, strengthening, and toning the body, and a good book to graduate to after making the initial commitment to embark on a fitness and health program. Spiral bound $11.95; paperback $9.95.

RUNNER'S WORLD INDOOR EXERCISE BOOK by Richard Benyo and Rhonda Provost. A simple-to-understand guide to fitness and the exercising body, and how it responds to beginning exercise programs, with programs keyed to the beginner and oriented toward getting started comfortably indoors before moving into outdoor fitness training and outdoor sports. Spiral bound $11.95; paperback $9.95.

RUNNER'S WORLD WEIGHT CONTROL BOOK by Michael Nash. A logical, realistic approach to losing weight and keeping it off forever that ignores the fad diets and gets right to the root of the problem: one's own image of self. A complete course in getting away from the multi-course meal. Spiral bound $11.95; paperback $9.95.

DANCE AEROBICS by Maxine Polley. The rage that has swept the nation. Getting in shape and staying there through an ambitious program of enjoyable, fast-moving dance that builds aerobic fitness while toning muscles and doing away with unwanted weight. Quality paperback. $5.95.

GETTING YOUR EXECUTIVES FIT by Don T. Jacobs, Ph.D. The book that America's corporations have been waiting for. A book that, in one package, reviews all available information on corporate fitness, while making the information accessible to everyone from hourly worker to chairman of the board. Large-format paperback. $12.95.